The

Gold

of the

Sunbeams

Also by Tito Rajarshi Mukhopadhyay

The Mind Tree: A Miraculous Child
Breaks the Silence of Autism

How Can I Talk If My Lips Don't Move?

The

Gold

of the

Sunbeams

and Other Stories

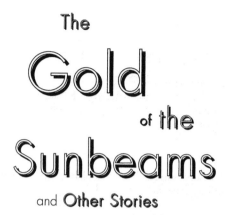

Tito Rajarshi Mukhopadhyay

Introduction by Soma Mukhopadhyay

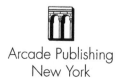

Arcade Publishing
New York

Arcade Publishing books may be purchased in bulk at special discounts
for sales promotion, corporate gifts, fund-raising, or educational purposes.
Special editions can also be created to specifications. For details, contact
the Special Sales Department, Arcade Publishing, 307 West 36th Street,
11th Floor, New York, NY 10018 or arcade@skyhorsepublishing.com.

Arcade Publishing® is a registered trademark of Skyhorse Publishing, Inc.®,
a Delaware corporation.

This is a work of fiction. Names, characters, places, and incidents are
either the work of the author's imagination or are used fictitiously.

Visit our website at www.arcadepub.com.
Visit the author's website at www.halo-soma.org.

10 9 8 7 6 5 4 3 2 1

Designed by API

Library of Congress Cataloging-in-Publication Data is available on file.

ISBN: 978-1-61145-253-2

Printed in the United States of America

Contents

Introduction

In 2001 my son Tito, who suffers from severe autism, and I came to the United States, when Cure Autism Now, an organization based in Los Angeles, California, invited us to take part in their research project. News of Tito's remarkable cognitive ability had reached America, and a number of neuroscientists from various universities wanted to study him to see if his progress could be transferred to others suffering from the same disorder. When I received the invitation, I thought, What a wonderful opportunity for Tito and me. America had always been the land of our dreams, and here we were sponsored to go to Los Angeles for four months! These four months would be, I was sure, the most valuable and meaningful period of our life. We were eager to learn, eager to experience. In Bangalore, India, where we were then living, we had a small, cramped apartment without running water. If nothing else, I thought, for the next four months we would be blessed with all the water we wanted!

When Tito was still very young, I had begun to realize that he had serious problems: he was locked behind a barrier of silence. At first, I had no idea that the problem was autism, nor that the prognosis was so devastating. I took him from one doctor to another, trying to discover what his problem was, to no avail. All I was told was that he was "mentally retarded," until finally he was diagnosed as severely autistic. Not only was he incapable of relating to others, but I saw that he had little or no control over his motor activities. Therefore he had to be closely and constantly supervised to make sure that when he was with others he did not embarrass himself socially. I was told he would never learn to read or write, or even understand. Yet I detected early on, from many of his reactions, that he seemed to understand what I was saying. I made up my mind to test that conviction on my part by reading to him, both in Bengali and in English, explaining words and ideas as I went along, and soon I realized that his cognitive ability was good. From that I went to an alphabet board, to teach him to spell. Using it, he began to respond to questions — pointing out, letter by letter, his responses — and later to answer by writing. In reading further, I decided to focus on English, because of its universality. I had begun teaching him when he was only three and a half, and by the time he was six — doubtless imbued with the stories and plays I had been reading to him over the years — he was writing himself. At first I had to fasten a pencil to his hand, but soon he was writing without being thus restricted. At eight, he had begun composing stories and poems of an amazing insight and complexity for *anyone* his age. For the next three years he continued to write, and by the time he was eleven he had more than enough material for a book. That book, entitled *Beyond the Silence,* was published first in Britain by the National Autistic Society. Later, in America and other countries, a longer version, incorporating many of Tito's new poems, was published under the title *The Mind Tree,* giving hope to autistic children around the world, and leading to our invitation to come to America.

As Tito's tests progressed, we learned more and more about this remarkable country and its people. Every aspect of our new life in America was a wonder: The running water. No power cuts. Clean, wide streets. What we saw of California impressed us to no end. Soon I was asked to teach other autistic children, using the method I used with Tito. Although I was sure of my work, I did not know whether it would be effective with children new to my unusual Indian dress and my accent. Before long, however, the results were so positive that I was working long hours every day, having been given a year's fellowship by Cure Autism Now to use my Rapid Prompting™ Method in a school for autistic children in Los Angeles. While working at the school I also focused on my larger mission: using my teaching method to reach out not only to children but also autistic adults throughout the United States.

In January 2003, *60 Minutes II* featured Tito, me, and my work, as a result of which I was invited as a keynote speaker at various conferences and to conduct workshops around the country. Other children not involved in my school began coming to see me at my home for instruction and guidance, on Saturdays, Sundays, and after school on weekdays. After the children were gone, Tito continued to study and write under my guidance. I suddenly realized, however, that I was working 365 days a year, including Christmas and New Year's! I decided I needed to slow down, to do justice to Tito, my health, and my mission. When in December 2003 I fell ill, I realized I could no longer handle all the clients — by that time some 300, ranging in age from four to sixty — clamoring for my services, hoping against hope that I could do for them, or their children, what I had been able to accomplish for Tito. The problem was, they lived all over the United States, and often they would call me, forgetting the difference in time zones, in the wee hours of the morning. Something had to change.

I called some of my clients-turned-friends and asked for their help. My work needs organizational help, I said, and I need some days off. I also need a paycheck that will support Tito and me. One who immediately and generously responded was my friend Linda Lange, who had a nonprofit organization called HALO — Helping Autism through Learning and Outreach — in Austin, Texas. I had earlier gone to Austin at her invitation — in fact just after September 11, 2001, for I remember how empty and desolate the airport was — and after my work there Linda handed me an envelope. I didn't open it then, for I don't feel it's proper to open payment envelopes in front of the donor. But when I got home and did open it, I saw an amount so far above my expectations that I called Linda immediately and said I thought she had made a mistake. "No," was her response, "it's only what you deserve."

Anyway, when I called her two years later, not only did she offer to support my work, she also said she would arrange to have someone prepare my schedule, which was taking too much of my time and attention. Further, I would have two days off every week, and have a decent salary to support us in our new country, some of whose ways were still foreign to us.

My work with HALO began in January 2004. While I was working at my clinic in Burbank, Tito went to a private school, where teaching nonverbal autistic students meant keeping them occupied with various activities and managing their behavior. I was constantly worried about Tito, for he was capable of so much more, but there was no other viable option. Still, without my presence and prompting, I could sense he was drifting away, although he continued to write in the evenings. But for his sake, I knew, we would have to find a better solution, which probably meant moving. But to where? The answer was evident: Austin.

When we arrived there, I was immediately struck by how much it reminded me of Mysore, India, where Tito and I had lived from the time he was five until he turned eight: the parks and trees, the university, the climate. So thanks to Linda Lange, we are now ensconced in Austin, working with HALO, and looking forward to the next stage of our lives, and to Tito's continued efforts to write more and more of the tales with which his fertile mind seems endlessly filled.

Soma Mukhopadhyay

The
Gold
of the
Sunbeams

The Showers

This was written when I was still in India. As I watched the news and saw pictures of a cyclone's aftermath, my heart went out to those brave people in the state of Orissa who suffered most that year. Resources were limited and help was not enough. So I created my own characters through my imagination to show my admiration for the people in that part of the country.

There was rain, a lot of rain that June. As if the whole month had been drenched with water. And the water had kept a hold on everything. The rice fields, the muddy roads, the pond where Kedar and Abu go to swim in the morning and where Kedar's mother, Suman's aunt, and Kariman and Abu's sister come during the afternoons to wash and chat and argue amongst themselves, the cleaner looking buffaloes, the banyan tree that stands in the centre of the village and around which the village has grown, the cemented platform under it, where old Mahim sat during those dry mornings to chat with Kedar's grand-father, Abu's sister's father-in-law and other old folks, all were equally drenched. The platform had become very slippery to walk or even sit on.

The crows that lived in the village had been quieter, per-haps because of the rains.

☼   ☼   ☼

"How much water can the sky hold?" Abu had wondered, looking at the sky. It looked as if all the waters of the earth had collected in the clouds just to pour on their village.

"The sky can hold everything," Kedar had explained to Abu. "Can't you see that it can hold all those stars, the sun, the moon, and even the whole of the heavens? I heard that all the dead people who become ghosts also go up there to stay in the sky."

Kedar was very satisfied with himself for being able to explain to Abu the power of the sky.

"And don't you see that even the gods stay up there?"

Kedar felt there was quite a logic in his words.

"Sometimes Abu asks such silly things!"

They were sitting on the bamboo platform by the river embankment, where Gopal and Viru come in the mornings to catch fish. The fishermen were not there that evening because they had gone to the town to sell the fish. So Kedar and Abu had got the whole platform to themselves.

Abu threw a stone in the muddy water of the river.

The river had risen high because of the flood. It was full of a great amount of silt, which would make the land very fertile later.

Kedar threw the next stone. They watched the ripples form and then be replaced by the ripples of the flow.

✻   ✻   ✻

The west side of the village was flooded.

The school was closed now for the time being. How could any school run when it was housing fifteen families? Fifteen flood-affected families. Fifteen families had made the school building their new home. Their homes were under the water. Where else could they go?

"Where should we go?" Dasu had asked Ganga Kishore, the headman of the village. "Yes, where should we go?" they had asked Ganga Kishore, looking at the school building. The school building was the only building made of bricks apart from Ganga Kishore's house.

They had all moved in the school building, with their babies, with their women, with their little bundles of belongings and their water pots and cooking pots and their young boys. They had also brought their buffaloes with them, but because the school headmaster had protested about their entry into the school building, they had been forced to tie the animals outside. The animals had given a longing look at the building.

A problem arose when every family wanted to occupy the headmaster's room. And since, that had led to a greater problem because to occupy that room, everyone needed to push the other one out, and someone was constantly getting hurt, so it was decided that the headmaster's room would be converted into a common kitchen. But the headmaster was throwing tantrums.

He would resign.

Finally, he agreed because the headman, Ganga Kishore, had given his word that he would get the room repainted if any scratch appeared on any wall.

"Where should we get our rations from?" Karim's wife had asked. Surely the grains could not be saved while they were saving their belongings.

She was scolded by her husband. "Woman, why do you talk when men are doing our talking?"

However, since the question was already raised, some answer was expected.

Certainly the answer could not be expected from Abu's sister's father-in-law or Haridas the moneylender, or from the farmers who were all staring at Ganga Kishore for some answer.

Abu had gone there.

Kedar had gone there.

Atul, Shankar, and even Shankar's three-year-old brother had gone there.

Of course, Tulsiram, Haridas, the moneylender, Abu's sister's father-in-law, Kedar's grandfather, old Mahim, and all the elders of the village had gone to the courtyard of Ganga Kishore.

Animals came too. Kedar had brought the goats of Mia Chaudhary, which he took out for grazing with him. He could not leave them on the field to graze on their own. Could he? Only last month Ratan's black goat had been found missing. Ratan was sure that somebody had stolen it.

"How could you leave your goat to graze all alone like that when half of the village is starving?" Ganga Kishore had asked him back. "You cannot blame anyone now if your goat happened to get cooked by some hungry family."

Surely no one could be blamed when the stomach was hungry and food was left unguarded. Since then Mia Chaudhary had been more careful about his goats. He had hired Abu and Kedar to look after them.

The highway which links the village to Karimgunj, the only town close by, was closed now because of the rising level of water. Even the railway track was now underwater. So Banwari refused to bring the supplies from Karimgunj in his trekker, which he fondly called his "car," because he said that the engine would get damaged if it had to be ploughed through the water.

"Where is the road?" he had asked back when they were willing to pay him for the trip.

"Then how should we get the supplies?" they had asked.

They had all assembled in the courtyard of Ganga Kishore. Men, boys, and animals. The women and girls came too but remained at a distance. How could they come forward when there were so many people sitting and deciding so many important matters? They were present, with their infants in their arms. They made their presence with their whispers, they made their presence with their bangle tinkling sounds, and they made their presence with their soft giggles here and there, now and then and again.

Everyone however waited for Ganga Kishore to speak.

Yet everyone had questions to ask.

"How should the supplies come in if Banwari refuses to bring them on his trekker?"

"Who should feed the fifteen families put up in the school?"

"What about the buffaloes?"

Questions were getting interrupted by more questions.

"Don't talk together." Requests were made.

"Why shouldn't we?" Requests were questioned back.

Kedar watched the men talk.

He watched the men. He watched them questioning. Questions like the raindrops turning down to the earth for their answers. And the earth, answering all of them back by flooding the village so that they could get reflected through the water. What can be a better reply?

He looked at the cloudy sky once again.

"Will the clouds ever move away from here?"

The clouds had looked back at him in such a way that he knew that even the sun would not dare to show its face to the village today.

✳   ✳   ✳

A goat had tried to move into the place right in front of the meeting, right in front of Ganga Kishore. Kedar ran forward to chase it back. And then he got noticed.

"Come here, boy," Ganga Kishore called him. Kedar looked around him. Surely it could not be him. But Ganga Kishore was looking at him.

He walked reluctantly near the headman. Headman was the headman, after all.

"This boy here will look after your buffaloes. The buffaloes will live here in my outside garden and this boy will look after them."

The headman announced it as if he was honouring Kedar with a big award. Kedar stood there by his side and obediently nodded.

He hated buffaloes.

Ganga Kishore was applauded. He had solved one problem. Ganga Kishore gave a polite smile back.

Kedar would ask Abu to help him manage those buffaloes. He knew how stubborn buffaloes were.

The other problem remained. Supplies.

Ganga Kishore started his speech.

"The need at present is to survive till the roads are opened once again. Viru and Gopal can take their fishing boats to Karimgunj and bring kerosene, rice, and vegetables. Till then, children below eight and elders above sixty will get two meals, while the rest of the village will have a meal before they retire to rest at night.

"There will be two common kitchens. Your wives and your elder daughters will volunteer. Food will be cooked by Ratan's wife, Kedar's mother, and Gopal's widowed sister for the Hindus. Karim's wife, Abu's mother, Mia Chaudhari's wife, and Amiran will cook for the Muslims.

"The Hindu meal will be cooked in the headmaster's room in the school. The Muslim meal will be cooked just outside my courtyard in front of my stable.

"And my wife will supervise everything because the supplies will go from my house."

Ganga Kishore felt good about his speech. He usually felt good when he was looked up to.

He needed to win the September elections. Only then he could get a permanent ticket in the Congress Party. He had heard from a source that the party was thinking of putting up a Muslim candidate that year. It would give the party a very secular image.

He also knew that Mia Chaudhary had his plans to contest the elections. He had seen Mia Chaudhary coming out of the party office when he had visited it last month. And Mia Chaudhary had hurried away when their eyes had met.

Ganga Kishore was waiting for an opportunity to impress people.

"What could be a better opportunity other than this flood?"

Mia Chaudhary was sitting at the back with narrowed eyes watching him.

Ganga Kishore was concluding his speech.

"As your headman, I feel responsible. And because I feel responsible, I take charge of all your plights. Feel free to come to me with your problems."

"Rascal!" Mia Chaudhary hissed out.

It had been a long day for Amiran.

She had helped the women cook the meal throughout the day. She had brought water, she had carried the wood, she had served the meals, and then she had cleaned up the place. She was tired. The other two women had already left, leaving her to put the things back in place inside Ganga Kishore's stable.

There were heavy pots to be lifted and carried from Ganga Kishore's courtyard to his stable, where once upon a time Ganga Kishore's father used to keep real horses. Ganga Kishore's wife would not have those vessels inside her house or inside her kitchen. How could she? The meal for the Muslims was cooked in those pots. No, she could not have those pots inside her kitchen.

Ganga Kishore never interfered in the petty household matters. So he kept quiet. He usually kept quiet when his wife showed her determination.

Amiran arranged the pots one by one so that it got easy to take them back to the courtyard the next day.

"Who knows when the fishermen will come back with fresh supplies."

Amiran was tired. She sat on the pile of dried wood on one side of the stable. She looked around.

"Imagine, there were real horses living here once."

Amiran had seen horses only once in her seventeen years of life.

Year before last, when the circus had come to Karimgunj, she had gone with Kamala, Kedar's mother, Ratan's wife, Abu's sister, and Abu's sister's mother-in-law to see the circus. She had seen many animals whose names she had only heard of before.

She had seen lions, elephants, and tigers there.

And she had seen horses.

She had envied that pretty girl who was doing tricks on the back of the horses.

"And how she dared to jump from one horse back to another!"

Amiran had dreams of horses and that daring circus girl for many days. And here she was sitting in the stable of Ganga

Kishore, where once upon a time real horses used to live. She sat on the dry logs and closed her eyes. Then she imagined those logs to be horse backs. She kept two logs side by side and began to jump from one log to another. "Just like that circus girl."

The door opened silently. And silently someone entered.

The door closed once again.

Amiran turned to see who the person was. She could not make him out because of his covered face.

The suddenness of the moment was too overwhelming for her. She forgot everything. Everything about the circus girl, everything about the horses, everything about getting back home, and everything about screaming out her fear and scream-ing away the man. She was waiting to be told what to do.

The man had placed his forefingers on her lips. She should not talk, let alone shout.

She did not shout. The scream had frozen to silence somewhere inside her. She heard her own silence screaming within her, knocking her down.

"Sit down, good girl."

The man had hissed a whisper.

She sat down, waiting to be told what to do.

For a while she had nothing to do. She had only to wait.

She had to wait for everything.

She had to wait for the man to go and take with him whatever he wanted to take, including his heavy, tobacco-chewing breaths and the suffocating smell of his sweat.

Amiran was left alone again with the logs and those cooking pots she had arranged moments ago with playful cheer.

There was nothing to be done anymore. Nothing for her to think. Nothing to play with.

All her screams now came out from her through her tears. No doubt those tears were too loud for her to bear alone in that dark stable of Ganga Kishore, the headman.

She walked out of the stable. Her teardrops got mixed with the raindrops.

"How much water can the eyes hold?" Amiran had wondered as she walked out and away from the stable, to anywhere. She would not go home. She would go anywhere till the last drop of nothingness seeped out of her eyes. And the nothingness in her saw that she could do so.

Stories formed.

Stories formed on the water-filled ground of the village like clouds forming on the stretch of the sky over the village.

Those stories got mixed up with the raindrops as they met somewhere in between the sky and the ground, where

Munira's aunt was telling Ganga Kishore's wife that her niece Amiran did not return home last evening.

And Ganga Kishore's wife had formed the first story since then. A probable story. How else could she form a story if she had not considered the probability?

"Did you check the whole village?" she asked Munira aunt. She was worried about the help in the cooking of the Muslim meal.

"Are you sure that Amiran did not run away with anyone? You see, her age is so delicate."

Ganga Kishore's wife laid the first foundation to the story.

As the day grew and people began to know about Amiran's disappearance, there were more stories to be formed around her. Some people were sure that they had seen someone jump into the flowing river in the middle of the night, when the rain made the loudest moaning sound. However, they did not interfere because they thought that it was the spirit of Lochan's sister trying to frighten them again three years after her death.

Every discussion got collected from scattered isolation. They got collected in the courtyard of Ganga Kishore.

Ganga Kishore sat in the centre and listened to everyone. He looked around at everyone and he heard every story from everyone. Every story looked back at him as he chewed the tobacco. Stories looking at him with expectations. Expectations collecting to form questions.

"What should we do now?"

"Where should we find her?"

"And who should go and look around?"

"Should someone go to Karimgunj and complain to the police?"

"What about the midday meal?"

All the raindrops collected around the stable where Ganga Kishore had seen Amiran play with the logs last evening.

He tried to collect the answers to every question. All his answers got gathered into a nod.

He nodded when Atul Maji asked him whether he should take his boat out to see if any dead body could be seen floating downstream.

He nodded again when Tilak Mandal and Ghias ud din volunteered to go to Karimgunj and file a police complaint.

And when Samar Khan proposed that he could send his wife to replace Amiran, for the time being, Ganga Kishore had nodded again.

He felt responsible during such moments. The whole village had looked up to him.

After all, he was responsible.

*   *   *

More water flowed and more stories flowed.

Gopal and Viru, who had gone to Karimgunj to buy the resources, had come back. Kedar and Abu had spotted them
first, when they had taken those goats and those buffaloes to
graze on the large mound on which the Sun God was believed
to come down on the earth once every year during summer
solstice, to assure the earth that he would continue to shine
down till life no longer existed.

So, during every summer solstice, there is the great Sun
Fair around the mound. It is attended by people from all the
neighbouring villages. Once there was a gypsy camp too. It
was then that Kedar had made up his mind to grow up to become a gypsy.

The mound is left to the cows and goats to graze on for
the rest of the year. Abu and Kedar had brought those goats
and buffaloes with them to graze. They had also brought some
puffed rice along with them to share and eat. They would automatically realise when they grew up that they were not supposed to share any food because they prayed to different gods.

At present they were sharing the puffed rice under the in-
exhaustible stretch of clouds. The rains had stopped since
morning. It was then that they had spotted the boats of Viru
and Gopal trying to plough their way around the submerged

trees, around old Giridhari's hut, whose roof was the only thing which was out of the water, perhaps waiting to get drowned too, like the walls, because Giridhari had taken shelter in the school building. They saw the boats finding it difficult to get through the place where Giridhari had planted a wire mesh fencing to prevent the goats from entering the garden where Giridhari had grown the night jasmines and merrygold.

They breathed relief when they saw the men slowly removing the wire mesh and throwing it far away, and then finally getting closer to the village.

Abu and Kedar wanted to run back to the village and see how the distribution was taking place. They wanted to see who got those white radishes and who got the leaves.

But they could not go leaving the animals there.

So they just watched the boats drift slowly away.

They watched the men slowly pushing the boats when they got caught by one of the pumpkin creepers of Madho Singh.

Kedar and Abu waved at the men.

Viru and Gopal were too busy to look up. To look up at the mound. The Sun God's mound.

Mia Chaudhary was standing on his rooftop with his hands folded, looking around at the fields. The water looked very muddy all around. One or two days more of the standing water, and all the paddy crop would get destroyed, and all the hard work would go to waste.

Mia Chaudhary stood there with a frown. He was concerned about the hunger, which would not spare the village after this. He knew that he would not starve. Nor would Ganga Kishore.

He was concerned about Moti, Ramsevak, and Taj ud din, who had worked day and night in his field. He was concerned about their children. He looked up at the sky once again.

He remembered how the village had run into a festival when the first clouds of the monsoon had flown into their village. He remembered how he had distributed sweets to all those who worked in his fields. Happiness and hope had come in with the clouds. He had announced a bonus if the crops grew well.

Hopes and dreams were followed with hard work.

The water had entered gradually and slowly, giving everyone time to get prepared. Nothing was drowned. People had enough time to move their pots, beddings, old men, animals, and babies.

Mia Chaudhary looked at the school building. He had sent his men to supervise the quarrels taking place there between the families.

Just then he saw Banwari running towards him. At first he pretended not to see him and tried to look surprised when he was near enough and their eyes met. However he kept his hands folded as before. Banwari had campaigned for him in the last elections when he had stood as an independent candidate. He was sure that if Banwari supported him this time all the people belonging to his caste would support him also. All he needed now was a Congress Party ticket.

"What is the matter, Banwari?"

"The fishermen have come back with the rice and vegetables. But their boats have been looted by some desperate villagers. They were beaten up when they tried to save the boats. Gopal's and Viru's arms were broken."

Banwari took his breath.

Gopal and Viru got some treatment for their broken arms. Certainly no one could expect any doctor to treat their arms. "Where can anyone find any doctor in this village, specially when the water has entered?"

Nobody could expect a doctor to come from the town just for the sake of the broken arms of two fishermen.

They were brought inside Ganga Kishore's stable. They could stay there, with their wives and children, for as long as it them took to recover.

Meanwhile, Ganga Kishore would try to do some justice. He promised to find those who were responsible for their broken arms and punish them. He was sure that those men had been sent by Mia Chaudhary. So he was certain that Mia Chaudhary would bring more harm to the village if he was given a Congress Party's ticket for the coming elections. He even gave a speech in his courtyard by calling the villagers.

"Surely everyone needs to be cautioned about Mia Chaudhary."

Gopal and Viru sat on either side of his chair. He spoke on how Mia Chaudhary should be stopped before he got out of control.

Kedar and Abu also attended the meeting, with the goats and buffaloes. After all, Viru and Gopal were their friends. They even looked after the fishing nets when Viru and Gopal went down the bamboo platform to have tea.

"Imagine Gopal and Viru sharing the same platform with the headman."

"They should be feeling very important sitting there," Abu whispered as he waved at Gopal and Viru.

"They did not see you." Kedar waved harder.

One of the buffaloes called back, not realising that the headman was in the middle of his speech.

"Take them away." Ganga Kishore looked irritated.

So they had to leave the meeting halfway through, because they knew that the buffalo would not shut up even if requested to.

Gopal and Viru continued to sit on either side of the headman.

The headman continued to talk and caution the villagers about the hidden enemy who had the most friendly smile.

Gopal's pain in his arm was growing, while Viru's arm had started to feel numb.

Someone had treated their arms with a paste of lotus stem and tamarind. They had not objected.

Arguments can take place any time and at any moment. And arguments can grow big depending on the intensity of those voices, which are actually taking part in it.

So no one was surprised.

Viru had complained of feeling the numbness in his broken arm and Gopal had complained of the growing pain in his. Kiran's mother had argued, "How can that be possible when the ailment is the same and the medicine prescribed by her is also the same," and when Abu's sister's mother-in-law replied back to her, "You don't know anything," no one was surprised that it was the beginning of an argument.

✻   ✻   ✻

Naturally when the argument was taking place in front of Ganga Kishore's stable, where Gopal and Viru were staying with their families and where they would stay till the floods remained, everyone had come to watch.

Viru's wife called Ganga Kishore's wife, because being the wife of the headman she ought to know what was going on in front of her stable. Ganga Kishore's wife called her best friends, Prasad's mother-in-law, Chaman's sister-in-law, and Durgadasi, her own widowed sister-in-law who stayed next door.

"Ask them to hold on till we come," she told Viru's wife, because she did not want to miss out on the most important parts of the quarrel.

Nobody wanted to miss out on anything.

So by the time she had gathered there with her best friends, there was already a crowd around Viru and Gopal, who looked rather embarrassed.

They tried to shrink their bodies as more and more women started gathering around them. They bent their heads, they crossed their arms and legs and sat close together with bowed eyes.

Abu and Kedar had heard about it from Ghias ud din. They stood with the group of boys and men at a distance. They could not take part, but at least they could hear. Why couldn't Abu be there when his own sister's mother-in-law was taking the lead? And if Abu could be there, why couldn't Kedar be? And if they could be there, why couldn't the buffaloes and goats be?

Kiran's mother was actually defending her prescribed ointment because she had heard that the paste made from lotus stem and tamarind was very good for bones. Specially broken bones.

And she had heard of it from none other than Ganga Kishore's own mother, who was now dead.

"And how can the headman's mother ever go wrong, especially when she is now dead?" She held a strong point there and challenged her opponent.

Abu's sister's mother-in-law had never expected such a strong point. But all the eyes had now turned towards her, and she knew that it was her turn to answer.

"How much tamarind did you put in that bowl of paste?" she demanded. That would teach the "loud-mouthed expert" not to outsmart her.

"And may we know why on earth the lady (may her soul rest in peace) chose you out of all of us to impart the knowledge of bone treatment?" Abu's sister's mother-in-law had a stronger point there.

"Yes, tell us why she chose to tell you and not us?" Ganga Kishore's wife echoed. She tried to give a sad look to show how much she missed her mother-in-law. It was much appreciated.

However, it was decided that Viru and Gopal would be treated by Abu's sister's mother-in-law for the next two days. If it worked, she would get two more days. If it did not work, Lochan's wife would give a try.

There were many people willing to try. Everyone would get a chance.

Everyone had come out to look up at the sky, including those who were staying at the school building, including old Bhoopi, who could not even move from one end of his room to the other end without help because of his arthritis.

However, today he did it entirely on his own, using his own willpower, because the sound which he heard from his rope-spun cot was enough for him to believe that the gods had come down with their rage to wipe out every trace of evil from the village.

They had all looked up. They saw the helicopter hovering around the Sun God's mound, where every year the Sun God comes down during the summer solstice in the disguise of a beggar.

Bhoopi realised that the helicopter was dropping food

packets and so it was flying as close to the ground as possible. Nothing should drop into the water.

It made a loud sound, and nobody could hear anybody, although everyone tried to instruct something or other to someone. Desperate instructions. Bhoopi also tried to instruct his son: "Get two packets for me also. Two will be enough for an old man like me."

Who knows who heard whom?

But everyone had started running towards the Sun God's mound. It did not matter who was running with whom now, but everyone tried to improve on their speed, especially when they saw others improving theirs.

So Ganga Kishore's wife ran along with her sister-in-law following close behind.

Mia Chaudhary ran close together with Ganga Kishore.

The marathon was over when the feet of young and old, women and children, had reached the Sun God's mound.

Packets were being dropped and packets were getting picked up. It did not matter how many packets got picked by one person. It did not matter who got pushed by whom in the process of packet picking. It did not matter to anybody that old Mahim was stamped by a frightened buffalo because the sight of so many people on the mound, the sound of the helicopter over their heads and the wind, which was blowing around because of the helicopter flying so low, was enough to frighten any buffalo.

Men, women, children, goats, and buffaloes ran together on the Sun God's mound.

Kedar and Abu had become hysterical. All the animals had gone beyond their control.

What should they do?

Abu started to pick up the packets. Kedar followed.

After all, the packets were meant to be picked up.

"What could have happened to Amiran?" Ganga Kishore's wife asked her husband.

The men who had gone in search of her came back without any news. But they had filed a case at the police station of Karimgunj and had filled out the forms giving her description.

The police had asked for a photograph. They could not show any because Amiran was never photographed before.

Some people are too ordinary to be photographed. And why on earth should Amiran be photographed when even Ganga Kishore's wife had never been photographed before in her life?

Ganga Kishore's wife explained to her husband while fanning him with the other end of her saree why she wished to be photographed. And how she wished to be photographed with her new necklace which was given to her by her father this year, and with the pair of earrings which Ganga Kishore's mother had possessed before her death, and which had automatically come down to her after her death because she had every right to them.

Ganga Kishore looked at the clouds and then at the end of his courtyard where the women were cooking the meal. Two days back, Amiran had been there to help. Ganga Kishore sat right here to watch her as she had bent down, as she straightened up, as she tried to check the big pot where the rice was getting cooked, as she played with the water that was kept in a bucket, as she dropped a few drops of water on the floor and as she joined those drops to make little drawings of stars and houses with water marks while she waited for the rice to get cooked.

Ganga Kishore thought how she had gone into the stable to bring more firewood and how she went there again to put the pots back in place at the end of the day. And then he remembered how he had followed her there and watched her play with the logs.

Ganga Kishore waved his hands to stop a fly from sitting on his nose. His wife continued to fan him.

"And don't you think I should also wear the bangles which you had given me last summer for my photograph to look effective?

"And perhaps I can have a photograph with you when you win the elections!"

Ganga Kishore's wife was planning to hang the photograph right in front of the courtyard. And surely Ganga Kishore would like to hang one in his office room.

How long was old Mahim lying unconscious after the helicopters had dropped the food packets? He had no idea. It was as if he were dreaming a long dream with the clouds, rain, and helicopter, everything included in the dream. He heard voices in that dream. And he heard buffaloes bellowing in that dream.

Everytime he heard buffaloes bellowing, he felt that his dream came to a halt.

And each time his dream halted, a pain flooded him, starting from his right chest.

Old Mahim tried to move. He could not. Then he tried to call out to his grandson. He could not do that either.

And all over again he started dreaming of clouds, helicopters, food packets dropping on the Sun God's mound, buffaloes running and buffaloes bellowing. Then once more he tried to call out to his grandson.

This cycle continued for some time, and slowly memory started to return back to old Mahim.

Seeing the helicopters dropping the food packets, he had rushed there too, along with the others. He had realised that he had really grown old when he saw others race past him to pick up the packets. When he finally reached the Sun God's mound, most of the others had already reached it. Many had collected at least six or seven packets. Desperate as he was, he did not realise that there was a buffalo running right behind him.

And then he just cannot remember what happened after he stretched out his hands to pick up a packet that was right in front of him.

He tried once again to spread his hands. All he could feel was pain.

"Drink this, Uncle Mahim." He heard a voice.

He heard the voice of Ganga Kishore in his in-between state of sleep and wakefulness. He could not open his eyes. However, he could open his mouth a little. Ganga Kishore fed him a spoonful of milk.

Old Mahim drank the milk and opened his eyes for the last time to bless Ganga Kishore. Yes, he was thirsty.

And then he closed his eyes once again, forever to continue with his eternal dream, which was larger than the beyonds of those clouds, the Sun God's mound, and the Sun God.

✻   ✻   ✻

Ganga Kishore held the hands of the dead man, as his grandson had been sent to Karimgunj to persuade a doctor to come to the village and treat him.

On the fifth day of the floods, Ganga Kishore went to the town to bring the district administrator to come and inspect the village and get some grants for the rehabilitation of the families whose homes have been destroyed by the floods. A great opportunity to show the villagers how much he cared. Only then would he get their votes for the coming elections.

The district administrator was reluctant to come at first. After two days the chief minister was to visit the office. How could he leave his office now? Couldn't anyone understand how important the chief minister's visit was and how busy his office?

However, he had assured Ganga Kishore that he would recommend Ganga Kishore's village to the chief minister. Of course he would make stronger recommendations if Ganga Kishore paid him something worth remembering, so that the name of his village would not escape his mind.

Ganga Kishore knew about it. He had come prepared already. He had brought two hens from his poultry. After all, the next election was close by, and he needed to impress the villagers. Only then could he win. And if he won he would get a permanent seat in the Congress Party.

✳   ✳   ✳

Assurances were exchanged with two hens. And smiles were exchanged. Ganga Kishore was offered tea when he promised to gift the officer two percent of the sanctioned money if the chief minister granted any.

Understanding was mutually exchanged.

Ganga Kishore came out of the office of the district officer. However, he met a familiar face waiting outside his room. The face belonged to none other than Mia Chaudhary. Ganga Kishore nodded at him, and Mia Chaudhary saluted back. Words were exchanged regarding their concerns for the homeless.

A goat called out from behind Mia Chaudhary. Only then did Ganga Kishore realise how similar their reasons had been regarding this visit.

"And the bastard has brought two goats to offer to the officer. Too smart for my two hens. And tomorrow I shall need to bring two more hens to make up for the difference," Ganga Kishore said behind his smile.

A silent smile.

"What do you think these buffaloes are thinking about all this water around the village?" Abu asked Kedar, looking at the peaceful buffalo faces.

"They must be too happy to spend their holidays with us," Kedar explained to Abu. He began to like them more now than before. "Why else do you think they carry us on their backs?" Kedar had a perfect reason to show why the buffaloes were so happy. "So what if they cannot laugh like us?"

Abu got a mild rebuke from Kedar for not understanding such a simple thing.

They counted the goats once again. There were two goats less because Mia Chaudhary had to gift them to the district administrator the day he went to Karimgunj to collect funds needed to feed the hungry people.

"But why are you taking those goats?" someone had asked.

"That is for the district administrator. Why should he give the funds if I don't give him anything?"

"Why should he need the goat? After all he would help us with the government money."

"Ganga Kishore has already taken two of his hens."

"You won't understand these complicated procedures in big offices." Mia Chaudhary assured them that hens don't work as well as goats work. "And remember those goats while you are voting for the coming elections."

He had to hurry now, as he knew that Ganga Kishore was already on his way to the district administrator's office with hens.

*　　*　　*

Abu and Kedar counted the goats once again.

"They could have fed the villagers with those hens and goats," Abu suggested.

"How could they pay the administrator if the villagers ate them?" Kedar argued.

Sometimes Abu gets such silly ideas that he has to wonder how to explain to him all the ways of life.

"But they could not bring the funds with them." Abu continued to talk silly.

"How could they bring?" Kedar was getting impatient.

"Didn't he promise that he would tell the chief minister?"

"And what else can be better than his promise?"

Snakes.

Snakes had started to come out on those places, which were being used by cattle and human beings, for living and cooking and sleeping. They were swifter than human beings.

Gopal's son had spotted one yellow and black ropelike thing behind the logs of dry firewood in Ganga Kishore's stable where his family was staying along with Viru's family. He had been very interested.

He had never owned any toy before. All he owned were his clothes, which he inherited from Mia Chaudhary's son, who had outgrown them. He also owned those round pebbles which he collected from the riverbed during those dry months. He made marbles with them. Sometimes he exchanged them with those green lozenges, which Abu bought from the shop belonging to his brother-in-law.

So when he saw the black and yellow snake in that semi-lit stable, he thought that it was some sort of a rope, which he could store in his box along with the stones. And then he could proudly show it off to his friends. He could imagine them envying him because of it. He would not allow anyone to touch it.

He made a move to pick it up. As soon as he bent down the whole pile of wood fell down over itself, rolling all over the stable. And the noise was enough to bring in all those who heard it. That also included Ganga Kishore's wife, who was supervising the cooking.

There was a "What happened?" expression in every face.

And when they saw the "What happened" in front of their eyes, more questions followed.

"How did it happen?"

"What are you doing alone in the stable?"

Gopal's son was feeling very nervous and embarrassed in the beginning. However, when the answers started coming out from him after Ganga Kishore's wife shook him up with great vigour, so that the answers could be shaken out of him automatically, panic started to spread.

"How big?"

"How thick?"

"Which colour?"

"Did it have a fat stomach?"

Many questions in front of Gopal's son to face them. How many questions were there in all? Gopal's son stood in the stable, suddenly realising how important he was.

"It was this thick." He gave a very thick measurement, spreading out his hands. The measurement should always depend on how important the question was. "And this long." He stretched his hands as far as he could stretch them, wishing that he could stretch them beyond that.

"A very fat stomach." He stretched out his hands again to show how fat the stomach was.

Once the measurement of the snake was understood, the colour of the reptile needed to be given so that everyone could be alerted.

"I think it was black and yellow. And perhaps a bit of red too." Gopal's son was not very sure about the presence of red on the scales of the snake. But he strongly believed that red would make the colour combination very effective. He wanted to add a little blue or perhaps a little green to it. But he stopped himself from that.

The description of the snake was more than enough to raise an alarm in the stable and in Ganga Kishore's courtyard.

Every log in the stable, every basket belonging to either Viru's family or Gopal's family, was dragged out. Every piece of blanket and every bit of rag was dragged out of the stable to search for the red and yellow and black reptile with a fat stomach.

Gopal's son felt very important. He was needed everywhere while the search went on to identify the snake. So sometimes he was needed in the stable, sometimes in the kitchen, and sometimes inside the house of Ganga Kishore. Otherwise who else would identify the red and black and yellow reptile? Gopal's son was quite impressed with himself.

The search continued. More and more talks went about. Talks about snakes. All those talks got collected together to form a ghost of fear in the village. Fear led to sleepless nights and dreaming of snakes in sleep.

Women in charge of collective meal cooking started to pay more attention to snake talks than cooking. An extra kerosene lantern was given to those who believed that any snake could be present in any dark corner.

But nobody could find the black and yellow and red snake that Gopal's son had spotted.

More reports came about someone spotting a green and blue snake in the school building, or someone else spotting an orange and white snake somewhere else. And because every new snake reported was turning out to be bigger and fatter than the previously heard one, there was every reason for everybody to talk of nothing else other than snakes. Snake seen last year by Sudhan's grandfather, which was as thick as a mango tree trunk, snake spotted near the pond near Madhu's rice field, which was as green as the rice plant and which Madhu had lifted up without recognising, thinking that it was a part of the plant, snake spotted at the roof of Mia Chaudhary year before last, and what about the one which Ganga Kishore's wife had seen on her bed the previous year?

Women chopped string beans, cautioning each other to be careful and not to chop any green snake disguised as a string bean.

"You never know how smart these snakes can be." Ganga Kishore's wife started to keep a bowl of milk day and night in places which she felt could be visited by snakes. She explained to other women that if snakes were fed with milk they would get intoxicated. And anybody should know that an intoxicated person is a happy person.

"Don't your men become happy when they are drunk?"

"So are the snakes." Ganga Kishore's wife definitely had a point there.

Some believed her, and as usual some did not believe her. Those who did not believe her started to light a fire around the places where they slept. Some tried to spot every hole on the walls and floors of their houses, and filled them with clay and stones.

And someone else called Sahabuddin, the snake charmer.

Chief minister had visited the village on the sixth day of the floods. He chose to walk on foot to survey the village, although Moti had offered to take him around on his bullock cart. Everyone had been concerned about his starched white clothes.

However, when he offered to walk around to prove that he was one with the people, "may it be flood or famine," everyone was impressed.

"Isn't he so humble?"

The officers who had accompanied him, however, did not seem to like the idea of walking in the dirty water. However they had no other option but to follow the chief minister.

Kedar and Abu had seen the procession progress from the Sun God's mound, where the buffaloes and goats were grazing with idle ease, not knowing anything about the importance of the chief minister's visit.

What impressed Kedar and Abu more was the awkward way with which the chief minister and his officers were walking on the water-filled fields. Each of them now losing his balance, then regaining it back, now falling and then getting up, now straight and then bent, now a jerk forward and then shaking back sideways, each step forward being more careful than the previous one.

Abu was getting concerned about them.

"What if we lend them a buffalo each to sit on?"

Kedar laughed aloud. Abu can really think silly.

"Why should a chief minister sit on a buffalo? That would make him look like Lalbabu the milkman. Can't you see the camera person taking his photograph?"

They could see both Mia Chaudhary and Ganga Kishore acting as guides to the chief minister's procession. Ganga Kishore could be seen pointing towards the northwest side of the village, while Mia Chaudhary could be seen pointing towards the southwest direction. The chief minister was looking down towards his feet, which were somewhere under the knee-deep water.

His shoe had gotten stuck somewhere. And when he tried to pull his left foot out, the foot had come out, leaving the shoe behind. There were many volunteers who dipped their elbows down in the muddy water to rescue the shoe. Chief minister's shoe. The camera person clicked.

It was difficult to locate the chief minister's shoes from the very beginning because the water was not transparent and was muddy. It resembled the colour of tea mixed with milk, from where Abu, Kedar, the goats, and the buffaloes were watching.

The men who were searching for the shoe looked more and more determined when, even after minutes had passed, the shoe was not recovered. They became more desperate when the camera person tried to take shots of them in the act. The water around them grew more and more muddy.

"Surely they are digging the ground believing that the shoe, in order to escape them, has gone underground."

Whatever could have happened to the shoe, time was running out fast. The procession started to move along towards the northwest side of the village. As the procession moved, it grew longer as more people joined it. Chief minister's visit was not something that could happen everyday. Especially when the chief minister was walking with the camera person.

Abu and Kedar decided that it was time for them to join the procession now. And why shouldn't they? When Gopal's son could join, when Mia Chaudhary's son could also join, why shouldn't they?

They started to descend the Sun God's mound.

They had to push the unwilling goats and buffaloes at first. However when the buffaloes understood what to do, they increased their speed all of a sudden, enough to alarm Abu and Kedar.

Two of the buffaloes were heading straight towards the procession. The goats, on the other hand, started to climb down all along the radius of Sun God's mound. None of the animals were paying any heed to all their shouts and instructions. Kedar was not sure how to collect them back. Abu felt that the number of goats was less when he counted them. He started counting them again.

On the seventh day, the level of water began to recede. It started to recede in the morning, and by evening it was only ankle-deep.

The chief minister's shoe could never be traced, and when he left, someone had given him a pair of rubber slippers to use. However, the chief minister's visit was very effective.

The village got a sanction with a relief fund which would be under the supervision of Ganga Kishore the headman. The chief minister became very popular with the women in the village after he posed for a photograph with them and addressed them as "My sisters and my mothers . . ." The camera person had promised to send a copy of the photograph when he developed it. Ganga Kishore's wife was already counting the days until its arrival.

She was very impressed with the chief minister's visit. She supervised the kitchen and thought about the chief minister sitting there on the courtyard where Ganga Kishore had laid a chair, his office chair, for the humble man. She thought about the chief minister drinking tea served by her sitting on "that chair," right "over there."

Although his tea was prepared by Viru's wife, she had snatched the cup from her hand and personally served the tea. The chief minister had complimented that it was the most refreshing tea he had ever had. And how it reminded him of his sister, who was the only person who had yet satisfied him with such kind of tea. Ganga Kishore's wife had blushed all along. However, she was disappointed with the camera person, who was more interested in taking shots of Gopal's son peeping from the stable. And then she realised that she should have known the simple fact.

"All camera persons are stupid."

Ganga Kishore's wife made plans for the group photograph when it arrived. She knew exactly what to do with it. She would hang it in her bedroom right in front of her eyes. And what if Kedar's mother or Abu's sister's mother-in-law or Mia Chaudhary's wife lay claim to it?

Her answer was simple.

She would not give.

The chief minister had won the hearts of the children. He had distributed sweets to them. And he even picked up Abu's sister's two-month-old baby, who had to dirty him at the right moment.

He became a hero for Kedar, as he did not mind when a buffalo misunderstood him and brushed its body with him while climbing down the Sun God's mound to join the procession.

*　　*　　*

It was the chief minister who had prevented Ganga Kishore from giving him a slap for the buffalo's conduct while he was trying to get the speeding animal under control before joining the procession.

Mia Chaudhary was surveying the paddy crops in his field. Water had completely left the village by now. There was no use keeping the crops because the lower parts of the stems were rotten due to the prolonged exposure to flood water.

He pulled out one plant and it came out of the soil very readily. He inspected the lower part of the stem. The blackened part told him that the colour would spread and engulf the remaining part of the plant with the infection.

He laid it on the soft ground with gentleness he could give as if the plant were someone very close to his heart.

He stood there alone looking at the destroyed crops with tenderness and regret. Hopes were destroyed. Hopes of Moti, Ramsevak, and Tajuddin were lying around destroyed at every stretch of the field. There was the stretching hunger waiting in front of the village. Now everyone would need to buy the rice which they could have sold.

Mia Chaudhary did not notice Moti, Ramsevak, and Tajuddin, the people who worked day and night in his rice field, standing behind him. Only when he turned around did he face them.

What could he tell them? They were waiting to be told something. Mia Chaudhary looked at the sun shining once again on the sky.

He ordered his men, "Clear the field. Prepare the field for vegetables. I shall go to Karimgunj and buy the seeds."

Munira aunt had seen the sunlight fill up her courtyard. She was filled with a new hope. Perhaps her niece, Amiran, would come back any day, now that the water had left the village. Won't she tell her old aunt where she had been all these days? Won't she tell her once again all the stories about the circus girl jumping from one running horse to another?

She had asked Banwari, Mia Chaudhary's bodyguard, to find her out when he went to Karimgunj.

Banwari had promised.

Munira aunt was sure that Amiran would surely be found.

She asked Ganga Kishore also to find Amiran, and the headman had promised. Wasn't he now a friend of the chief minister?

Now she asked Mia Chaudhary.

He promised her he would do whatever he could.

Ganga Kishore had gone to Karimgunj to get Gopal's and Viru's broken arms treated. They were relieved because they were too tired of getting treated by Kiran's mother, Abu's sister's mother-in-law, and Lochan's wife.

All these days in continuous succession each one of them treated their broken arms with different paste. They had tasted the margossa-leaf paste and the turmeric paste. They had applied every composition of lotus-stem paste and turmeric on their hands. Yet they were too humble to revolt.

Their hands remained swollen all the same. And for the past few days the three women had been quarrelling so much that they had to take Kiran's mother's specially prepared margossa-juice tonic in the morning, betel leaf with a spot of honey and turmeric in the afternoon as recommended by Abu's sister's mother-in-law, and raw pumpkin with bitter-gourd-paste tablet at night.

So when Ganga Kishore offered to take them to a town doctor, they were more than glad.

Abu and Kedar were slapping the buffaloes back to the school building, where their owners would collect them.

However, when they reached the school, they saw something else. None of the dwellers who had made the school building their home was prepared to leave now. The headmaster was shouting at the top of his voice, asking everybody and ordering everybody to vacate the building as the water had now receded.

"Where should we live?" they asked.

Their homes were washed out by the floods. The ground

was still wet and too soft to rebuild their houses. "Maybe after a week."

"Nothing doing." The headmaster kept his volume loud.

There was every reason for him to slap the little boy who imitated his voice and said, "Nothing doing."

Mia Chaudhary had to stand by the common people and request from the headmaster a week's time. "Just a week and not a day more." He turned back, promising to return next week.

Only when he turned, he saw the buffaloes patiently waiting to be let inside the school.

"And not those animals." The headmaster was more determined.

Abu and Kedar had left the buffaloes at the school gate and so they could not hear him.

The sun shone brightly on the black backs of the animals, who were looking with admiration at their new home. The school building.

Just a Smile

Being autistic, the social smile is always difficult for me. But my under-standing and appreciation for smiles in faces is no less. This piece is a tribute to all your smiles.

The train had pulled us along with its old engine, which gave every sort of groaning sound, as if trying to tell everyone that it was time for it to retire.

The old man who sat in front of me with his legs crossed and ears covered with a muffler looked away from me when I gave him a smile of a "hello." Since I did not close my smile yet, I turned my smile at the lady sitting opposite my window on the other side. And since she had smiled back at me, the gentleman who was travelling with her had tried to shield her from my sight. He had given me a glare as if to tell me "dare and smile again."

I kept my smile for another minute or so and tried to re-ply "here I dare."

Just a smile. A very friendly gesture. It can turn events into favourable or unfavourable situations, depending on who you are smiling at.

Long long ago, when God was creating the everything, He must have smiled the first smile. He must have smiled at Himself, and so it has been unrecorded. He then passed it over to man, His favourite creature of the universe. Man began to smile since then through ages. Thus smile is a unique feature of man.

So I have never seen a smiling parrot or a smiling cat, apart from the picture of Alice's Cheshire Cat, who must have smiled in Wonderland.

How would a cow look if she did try to broaden her mouth and smile at a bull? My imagination gives up, and I looked out of the train window. Memories returned regarding that smile of mine which had created a big problem back in my school.

It was during one of my math classes. I was seeing one of my daydreams. So there was absolute peace within me because the math teacher, Mr. Sebastian, could not guess whether I was seeing the board or my dream. However, when he had asked a question looking at me, I knew it was time for me to wake up. And since I could not understand what he was talking about, he wanted to see my notebook, where I was supposed to take down what was there on the board. And it had happened then.

When Mr. Sebastian was in the process of throwing my math notebook out of the classroom window, the book had accidentally landed on the principal's head. How could Mr. Sebastian even guess that the principal would cross the path travelled by the notebook? And it was quite natural for me to grin, because Mr. Sebastian had made such an embarrassed face. Then in the process, my grin had grown broader, till my mouth had felt too small to hold that grin anymore. One thing followed another.

The principal's stepping inside the classroom, Mr. Sebastian's apologies, his pointing finger towards me, my faking a headache, my legs finally giving away to prove how weak I felt and Mr. Sebastian's disbelieving me because I was still grinning, the principal's calling me to join him at his office and I following him because there was no other option left for me. However I had to keep up my grin now on my face to prove that I had a very natural grin.

I suppose that the principal was not impressed with my smile, because I was asked to stay back after school and complete my incomplete work. No, he wouldn't listen to my appeal that I had a cricket match in the evening, even though I had invited him to watch it.

Out-of-place smile can cause a lot of problems.

Sister-in-law was visiting us last year. She had completed some degree in classical music. The location was my open terrace under a moonlit summer evening.

"Let us hear a recital," all had requested. I had requested, too, although I never can understand the complicated grammar of classical music. Sometimes when everyone says something and you don't it looks very unsporting.

Sister-in-law had fussed for a while. "Throat is giving trouble."

But since everybody encouraged her, I wanted to join in also.

"Come on, your voice is sweet enough to make the blood which is racing in and out of my heart increase the level of sugar," I had said. However I had to stop because my wife had given me a severe frown.

The song had begun.

A moonlit open terrace, a prime summertime, a handful of listeners, and a throatful of classical song.

Everyone had started to nod. Since everyone nodded I started to nod also.

Everything was going well, as it should. A classical recital and our heads nodding. However, there came an interruption. My next door neighbour, Mr. Sen, has an Alsatian named Ping Pong. Mr. Sen is sure that if Ping Pong was born a human, it could have developed a talent for music. And Ping Pong had proved it that day that it had some talent in this field.

So when Ping Pong heard the classical recital of my sister-in-law, it must have got motivated. Animal and plant lovers have proved this point some years back. They say that plants grow better when you play music to them. You cannot argue back about the location of their eardrums, because they are so sure. However when I heard Ping Pong being so appreciative about the classical recital, I had to accept the truth in the fact.

So every time my sister-in-law's pitch touched a particular note, Ping Pong gave a similar howl. Nobody had paid any attention to it for the first time. However, when it began to get repeated the next time and again the next time, I realised the dog's natural inclination towards music. Classical music. Sister-in-law's classical music.

Human beings are human beings. They can appreciate dogs barking and wagging the tails. But if a dog prodigy happens to appreciate a human being giving a classical recital, there is no doubt about some mixed feelings. Some may not accept the fact. My sister-in-law did not. In fact she was offended.

And when she saw me with my smile she had got up and had locked herself inside a room. And she wouldn't come out when we all pleaded with her that dinner was served.

My wife had apologised on my behalf because she was sure that it was not Ping Pong, but I, who was responsible for all this. I offered to apologise personally but could not do so because my wife had given me another glare.

However, Mr. Sen, who was one of the guests that evening, gave me the solution. "Ignore the problem." But ignoring the problem irritated my wife all the same. "How could you have dinner without waiting for us?" she had hissed out, looking at the locked door.

Later I heard that the sisters had dinner at midnight, long after I had fallen asleep. Hunger was the reason that day for my sister-in-law's opening the door and having the meal.

Perhaps one day my sister-in-law would forgive me for the smile. After all, just a smile.

"Perhaps one day man will understand that dogs like Ping Pong could have taste for music." Mr. Sen kept his hopes up.

"But Mr. Sen, dogs will never be able to smile, even if they wanted to," I had argued.

A smile on a man's face can be mysterious as well as revealing.

When I had asked a man in a red shirt sitting by the window of a bus, peeping out at the whole world, whether that bus would go to Lake Park or not, he had smiled the most mysterious smile. It could have meant anything. A yes or a no. I did not follow what his smile had meant. So I had asked my question again. The man in the red shirt repeated his smile. By then, the bus had started. My question followed it, leaving me standing there at the bus stop alone. I had to stand there for the next half hour or so.

My schoolday friend John would smile in a similar way whenever our geography teacher, Mr. Paul, would ask him something.

"John, can you tell me where the taiga vegetation is?"

John would answer with a smile.

"John, what are the people living in the tundra called?"

John would smile again.

"John, who scored the highest runs in the 1981 test cricket?"

"Sunil Gavaskar, sir." John would not smile this time.

The mystery of John's smile was revealed that day.

Some smiles can be very revealing.

Like the smile on the face of the vegetable seller who wanted ten rupees for a single cauliflower.

He knew that the cauliflower was chosen by me from the very beginning. I knew that it belonged to no one other than me. Some kind of bond between the vegetable and me.

A similar bond was felt by my wife, the other day, when she had spotted a red silk dress on the show window of a shop. Such bonds make you feel very possessive about those things.

As I was talking about the cauliflower, which was ten rupees, I knew that it had waited in some vegetable garden, then in some transporter's truck, and now on the heap with all those cauliflowers. It had waited all that time for me to buy it.

The vegetable seller had understood my hesitation to part with my ten rupees and my bond with the vegetable. The man had said nothing. He just smiled. He picked up the vegetable and turned it around right before my eyes. His smile had said it all.

"Some things are priceless."

There were no words exchanged. Just smiles.

My ten rupees, however, got exchanged with the cauliflower.

In movies, a dying man smiles, especially if he is a hero.

I remember the last scene of a movie which made my wife get so moved that she had started sobbing helplessly, making me embarrassed all the more.

The scene was a dying scene, when the hero was smiling a very peaceful death smile and his friend was weeping passionately by his side. My wife was so touched by the scene that she saw the movie three times after that.

She went with Ms. Sen.

Then she went with Ms. Sen and Ms. Sen's mother.

After that she went with Ms. Sen, Ms. Sen's mother, and Ms. Dixit.

Before she planned her fifth go, the film was gone.

Such was the smile of the dying hero.

I heard that the hero was awarded something later that year for that dying man's smile.

But a dying man's smile is not universal. When I had visited my boss's father's funeral, I did not see any smile on the face of the dead man.

✿　　✿　　✿

A smile is valuable. But its value is not recognised sometimes.

I had once tried to show my smile at the counter before paying up for my laundry. I had no change in my pocket. The man sitting at the counter was not ready to accept my five-hundred-rupee note. I knew however that he had the change notes in that drawer of his and did not wish to part with them. "I suppose the only solution is that you give me the service for free," I had suggested, giving my most friendly smile as a gift. He did not understand its value and he would rather pay me the change. So what else could he do other than open the drawer and give me the change.

The beauty queen won her crown by her "winning the heart" smile. Her famous smiling face can be seen any other day on any other page of any other magazine. A dream smile.

This dream smile caused some eyebrow raising at home because my wife did not like the idea of my reading about her so much. Her parents' view, her school principal's view, her hair designer's view, her photographer's view, her boyfriend's view, and everybody else's view.

Most of them knew when she was three that one day she would win the world with her smile.

I had to read them when my wife was not looking. I never expected her to understand the magic of a beauty queen's smile.

The smile on the face of one of our prime ministers. P. V. Narsimha Rao, was so rare that it was a photographer's delight if he managed to get a frame with his smile. And the smile of Mona Lisa. The million-dollar smile. All the hidden mysteries of the world included in that smile.

I thought of Mona Lisa. I thought of the beauty queen. I looked inside the compartment of the train again. I smiled at the old man sitting in front of me. He yawned back. So I continued my smile to offer it to the lady sitting on the other side of the compartment. She looked at the man who was travelling with her.

And when she was sure that the man was fast asleep, she smiled back at me.

For a while I could forget Mona Lisa and the beauty queen.

I smiled once again. And then again. The train kept moving.

The Gold of the Sunbeams

Thousands of young children in rural parts of India grow up without realising what it means to be educated. My father had described to me the village where he grew up. I had been there once or twice when I was young and when travelling was not so painful for me. (I am scared to travel long distances now because I get overwhelmed due to my autism.) I always wondered how it felt to grow up like the character Murali of my story did. It is a piece of my heart.

One

Murali had to go to the town the very next day. He had to go with Dayaram. And they had to leave for the town by the seven o'clock local train. Murali's father was in the police lockup. Murali knew nothing more. Neither did Dayaram, his neighbour.

Murali was left with a hut, a Grandmother, and a brother about half his age. Murali was not at all sure about his own age, although he had heard Grandmother talk about the floods when he was born. However, he considered his brother to be an infant.

His brother, Dasu, considered Murali to be a big man. And a man of their house. Man of the house indeed! For Murali had to draw water from the well early in the mornings with his thin brown hands, for Murali had to mix all those herbs in the right proportion for Grandmother's knee pain, for Murali had to make margossa-twig bundles for their father to sell in the train and in the town, for Murali had to cook and Murali had to wash, for Murali had to make those kites for Dasu with those coloured papers and then go to work for Chaudhary the landlord.

And because Dasu was still a child, Murali saw that he got the best share of the piece of pumpkin which Murali had cooked for dinner last night. And because Dasu was still a child, Murali cautioned Dasu every day to stay at home with grandmother while he was at work.

"Dasu, stay at home. You never shall know when the big fish will catch you if you go too near the pond.

"Dasu, stay at home if you want me to make you the red kite."

Dasu would obey this time. How he loved to fly a red kite in the blue sky! Red kite like a red dream. And what could be the red dream of Dasu?

You will never know. And you will never know because it is a big red secret of Dasu.

Murali had a secret too.

He waited to grow old. As old as Sunder and Babu. Only then he would be able to get thirty rupees a month. He tied his turban harder with greater determination, till his forehead refused to take more pressure.

And then all of a sudden he heard about his father being in the lockup. He would be there till God knew when. Why he was there was known only to God and Kashiram. And Kashiram had told nothing about it to Dayaram. How could he tell in such a hurry? He was a busy man, after all. He had to hurry to see his ailing father-in-law. But he had assured Dayaram that he would tell it all when he came back after two days.

Murali could not wait. And Dayaram assured to come along with him to the town and see Kirpal, his friend and Murali's father, by the seven o'clock train.

The night waited with them.

Two

They did not wait for Kashiram's return. They went the very next morning to the town. Grandmother had promised Murali that she would stay calm for the sake of little Dasu. Murali would, after all, return with all the information about his father. Even Chaudhary the landlord had promised to give Murali the loan if the police wanted money. The stationmaster too had promised to help.

Murali had not been to the town very often. Nor had Dayaram. So how should they know where the prison was? Dayaram asked the tea vendor who was selling tea in the same compartment. The tea vendor did not know. And all the other passengers sitting around did not know either. However, everyone wanted to know why they needed to go to the prison without getting caught.

"This boy's father is in the lockup since yesterday." Dayaram pointed towards Murali.

Curious eyes turned towards him. Murali looked down. Was he ashamed of his father? He was not sure. But the people around now started talking.

"I knew a family where the grandfather was a petty thief, the father was a pickpocket and the son turned to be a chain snatcher," a gentleman told Dayaram. Murali felt a warm drop of tear roll down his cheek.

"And what happened after that?" Somebody wanted the story to continue.

Murali got up. He stood by the door of the compartment. The breeze hit his face and dried up his teardrop. A mark remained. Dayaram stood next to him. After all, he felt responsible. He would not ask anybody anything about the prison anymore. At least not in a crowded train.

There was a little halt for a while. Murali directed all his thoughts towards one thought. Impatience. And he turned his impatient eyes towards Dayaram. "How long is the town from here?"

"Fifteen minutes," Dayaram speculated.

Both were hungry.

But money was too precious now for them to buy food. And both knew very well that they would not die if they skipped a meal. The police might ask for some money for allowing Murali to meet his father.

The train started moving. And the noise of the train assured Murali once again. Murali thought that it said, "Fifteen minutes, fifteen minutes, fifteen minutes . . . and fifteen minutes," with a continued echo, with his own heartbeats.

It continued to say "fifteen minutes" till the train reached the town and came to a halt.

Three

Murali counted his money. Rupees two, plus five, plus all those coins, made it nine rupees and eighty paises. He counted them once again. This time more carefully, hoping that it could become at least one or two rupees more.

Dayaram counted his money. Together both of them had thirty-seven rupees and twenty paises. They decided to tell those policemen who were standing at the prison gate and sharing the dry tobacco leaves amongst themselves that they had only twenty rupees in all. Who knows how much they would ask to allow them to meet Murali's father, Kirpal?

Dayaram kept the rest of the money safe inside his vest pocket. The policemen certainly would not find out.

"Clever Dayaram!" Murali appreciated.

However the policemen allowed them inside without questioning them. Murali was surprised. Dayaram was relieved. "And imagine people telling how the policemen bully you to take all your money!" Murali would surely make little Dasu a policeman when he grew up.

The big officer who sat on a chair spoke to Dayaram very kindly. Dayaram was also very polite with everyone. "We want to meet Kirpal Singh," he told the big officer, so politely that Murali wondered whether it was the same Dayaram who wins the trophies in the intervillage wrestling competitions. "And to think of it, he was the same Dayaram who can break a coconut on his own head!" Murali looked now at this humble Dayaram.

He looked at the thin constable who was leading them through the corridors of the prison.

It looked like a long wait. Kirpal came out at last through some lost corner of the corridor. "A being from another world." He wore a strange dress which the prisoners are supposed to wear.

But he returned to Murali's world when Murali finally heard him speak.

The charge against him was gambling in the park. Usually he managed to run away whenever he saw any police nearby. "Only yesterday, I was not lucky." Kirpal sighed.

"And imagine this! Yesterday I was winning for the first time."

Four

A lot needed to be planned. And a lot needed to be done.

The thin constable who had brought his father into that room to meet him had assured Murali that his father would not be there for more than two months.

And surely Kirpal Singh would not starve for those two months.

"For no one starves in a jail," Murali had assured grandmother, who would not stop worrying and weeping. "And no little boys go to jail, even to visit their father," Murali had to tell Dasu, who would not stop requesting Murali to take him there. "The policemen who stay there may lock you up."

And showers of questions followed from Dasu.

"Are those policemen very strong?"

"What do they look like?"

"Are their mustaches more curled than Dayaram's?"

"Are they taller than Chaudhary the landlord's body-guards?"

"What do they eat?"

Dasu refused to listen to anything else other than "policemen stories."

Murali exaggerated every answer of his. And he continued that every time Dasu fussed over his moringa-leaf curry and wanted to know why Murali did not cook anything else.

"Dasu, eat it up. Otherwise the policemen will come and catch you."

"Dasu, stay with Grandmother and don't go near the pond. You may not know where the policemen are hiding."

And a lot was needed to be planned. For Grandmother was out of funds and Dasu should not starve. Murali would sell margossa twigs in the train like his father did, till his father was out from prison. Later during the day, he would go to the landlord's farm. The landlord would understand why he was late.

Murali could be a bit late some days in reaching the farm. But the landlord would surely know that it could not be Murali's fault. For Murali had to do all those usual things which he did before. He had to cook and wash, he had to make bundles with the margossa twigs, and he had to do all those this and thats, including washing little Dasu, who was always filled with mud.

And of course, once a week he went to see his father in the prison. He could go alone. The thin constable turned into an absolute friend of his. Murali had offered him a bundle of margossa twigs the last time they met. Kirpal Singh looked more plump in the prison than elsewhere. Murali heard his father's future plans.

Kirpal Singh would join the Congress Party after his release. He would fight the *panchayat* elections. He could either win or he could not win.

If he won, he would be powerful. And if he was powerful, he would be rich. And if he got rich, this would be and that would be.

Time would pass with dreams. And dreams would grow to hope. Murali felt rich every time he came out of the prison after meeting his father.

"Once there was a rich margossa twig seller . . ." Murali began his story.

"Richer than a policeman?" Dasu asked.

Five

They usually live on the platform of the village railway station. Murali's village. They have their pots and their pans. They have their boys and they have their babies. They have their dogs, monkeys, and snakes. They have their tents and their strange language. They are gypsies.

Murali cannot understand their language. Nor does Kashiram, who goes nearly every day to the town to meet his father-in-law. Nor does Keshav Babu, the station master.

They talk and swear and they fight and sing in that strange language.

They also show monkey and snake tricks when a crowd gathers around them. Murali has seen a boy like him train a monkey, early in the mornings when he waits for his seven o'clock local train. He watches with all admiration when the monkey climbs up on a pole balanced on the boy's chest, as the boy arches backwards.

"How old could he be?" Murali wonders.

The boy ignores Murali.

The seven o'clock local train comes and Murali collects his bundles of margossa twigs. The train picks up speed. Murali looks out from the train window at the boy, who ignores the train.

"Wish I could be a monkey trainer." Murali sighs.

"Boy, give me a bundle of twenty," the first customer calls him.

And the day waits to be covered.

The ten o'clock local train would bring him back to his village. And then he would go to the landlord's farm. Yes, he would be hungry. But he knows that he would not die if he skipped a meal.

All depended on how you got used to hunger. And then when his father would come out and win the elections and get powerful and then get rich, he would again get used to some breakfast as before, when Kirpal had a job in the aluminum factory.

When Murali returns to his village, he cannot see the gypsy boy and the monkey anywhere around. Some women, some babies, some dogs, some pots, some quarrels, and some flies remain. "The men, boys, and animals must be in the next village."

Murali hurries to the landlord's farm.

Six

Kirpal thought of all those plans which were brighter than his prison cell. For only its darkness could show their brightness. And those bright plans kept his spirit filled with hope.

"I could migrate to the town and be a porter if I do not win the elections. Or I could sell vegetables. Perhaps I could be a broker in real estate in the city. Perhaps I could sell betel leaves." Perhaps and perhaps. Endless of all the perhaps.

Murali listened to all those dreams. And Murali added

more to them when he told them to Dasu, as the two brothers slept huddled together in their rope-spun cot.

Grandmother listened too. As she coughed and groaned in her blanket, giving deep sighs.

Dreams looked back at them through the darkness of the night, brightened by every assurance of possibility. Again during the daylight, the same dreams looked at them, darkened by the reality of hunger and toil.

Murali went in the morning to meet Kirpal. Dasu wanted to come along too. Murali did not take him. How could he? The town was filled with shine and glitters. Suppose Dasu asked for those green marbles? Or suppose Dasu asked for those orange or red ice candies which the man who stands outside the railway station sells? Murali would not be able to afford that. And Dasu would naturally get upset if he was refused. Murali still remembers how Dasu had become upset when Murali had refused to buy him the golden-coloured elephant doll in the village fair. Murali was upset too when Dasu would not understand.

On his way to meet his father, Murali was satisfied. He was satisfied because he could sell all the bundles of margossa twigs which he had that morning. And there was a full treasure with him. Fifteen rupees! And he knew that his father, Kirpal, would dream richer today.

Murali dreamt rich too. A dream worth fifteen rupees. The dream included some glass marbles for Dasu and grandmother's betel leaves with hazelnuts.

All those dreams got included in a bigger dream which Kirpal was talking about today.

"I will buy a cow!"

Seven

Cows can be a great nuisance sometimes. Especially when they are left to stray on their own. They just would not understand that Murali's Grandmother had planted that melon creeper only two months back and she was hoping it would flower any day.

So when Dayaram's cows, the black one and the white one, had a feast on the creeper, Grandmother had every reason to get upset about it. Although Dasu was happy because he hated everything about melons. He dared not show it in front of Grandmother. Dayaram was embarrassed about his cows' conduct. Only Dayaram's wife had justified the feast, saying that cows had a different sense of morality. "That makes them different from humans."

Problems needed solutions. And it was agreed that Dasu would take the cows every day out to graze. Both the cows.

The black one and the white one. In return, he would earn a midday meal in Dayaram's house. Dasu grabbed the opportunity. It would mean going out into the fields and flying kites with Mustaq and Rafiq. He did not show too much eagerness. It would make Murali restrict some of his freedom. "Murali is always like that."

Now no one should blame Dayaram if his cows stole the green *brinjals* from Bir Singh's vegetable cart. And Chaudhary the landlord would not blame Dayaram if his cows ate all his yellow merrygold from his garden. Dasu, too, would not be hungry. So when Kirpal would be released, he should not tell that his neighbour Dayaram had not looked after his son.

Dasu set off the very next day with the cows. He went off immediately after Murali had left for the station with those margossa twigs. However, Dasu wished that Dayaram paid him instead of giving him the meal. But he dared not utter anything for fear of losing his freedom.

"How about taking those cows to the pond for a swim!" Or, "Perhaps tie a kite on the white cow's horn!"

Eight

Chaudhary the landlord had called Murali in the afternoon after he came to work on his farm.

Murali waited with his bowed head in front of the big man. And the big man sat looking at Murali, on a broad wooden chair with a lot of cushions around him. Then he spoke.

"I am opening a school in my courtyard tomorrow. Send Dasu in the morning."

Murali nodded. How could he tell such a big man that Dasu had a job from morning till evening to look after Dayaram's cows? Where should Dasu find the time to come to a school? And wasn't coming to school a luxury, when stomach remained empty? What should Dasu do after getting educated?

Murali has seen people getting educated and going to town. They all end up being unemployed, because they all want to work in an office and become postmasters. To become a policeman, you don't need to be educated. The thin constable of the prison where his father is locked up had told him that he was not educated.

But Murali could not tell all this to Chaudhary. Wasn't he a big man? Didn't Chaudhary own a gun? Murali would rather talk to Dayaram. Dayaram would understand. And Dayaram was quick to understand. Although his wife was not so quick to understand. But Murali knew about it. "Women always take some time to understand."

But it was Dasu who just would not understand.

"They lock the boys in school."

"They don't even allow the cows inside."

"They beat the boys till their backs turn blue."

"I will never be able to keep my promise."

"I have promised the cows to take them for a race with the train."

Dasu refused to do anything with the school. He hated the landlord's son. He fought for his freedom till he was tired and everyone was tired. Even a policeman story would not calm him down.

Nine

Chaudhary's courtyard school. Chaudhary's new fancy. He would watch the little boys gather together in his courtyard, where his nephew Kumar would teach the first batch of his pupils.

And schools needed rules. Chaudhary made rules for his school also. The first rule was singing the National Anthem. Chaudhary would wave his hands, and the boys would close their eyes and sing the National Anthem.

Dasu pretended to sing too, although he did not know the words. Neither could he understand what the song was about. He thought about Dayaram's cows while he pretended to sing. If Murali had not frightened him, telling him about

Chaudhary's gun, he would have been out there with those animals.

But he was already here. In Chaudhary's school. He looked around him with curious eyes.

"So that is where Chaudhary's well is!"

"So that is where Chaudhary keeps his goat!"

Chaudhary sat comfortably with a half sitting and a half lying posture on a rope cot with very satisfied eyes. "What an opportunity of social work! A free school."

The scholars were proving to be a very difficult lot from the very beginning. Kashiram's son Raghav pushed Dasu. Dasu kicked back. Soora took Dasu's side, while Rafiq took the side of Raghav. And the silence was turning into grunts and groans. Chaudhary frowned. When he frowned, Kumar the teacher became alert. The second rule of Chaudhary's school was discipline.

So Kumar looked at Chaudhary for an approval before punishing Raghav and Dasu. Raghav was asked to kneel, and Dasu was asked to stand on one leg.

The rest of the class recited the vernacular alphabet after the master. Each boy fiercely shook his head as a rhythm formed on its own. Chaudhary dozed. Dasu balanced on one leg.

"What are those cows doing now?

"Wonder how long the school will continue."

Dasu was hungry. He remembered Dayaram's wife had cooked the coconut curry last morning. And he longed to be a cowherd once again. Tomorrow he would fake a headache and remain at home while Murali was still there. After that he was sure that Grandmother would not run after him with her knee pain.

Dasu brightened up with a wonderful idea. "Why not pretend to faint now?"

Kumar was nervous and Chaudhary was frightened. Students were confused. Who would ever be prepared for Dasu to faint? Dasu could hear a great confusion around him. Chaudhary did not have any idea what to do. Dasu allowed them to carry him wherever they wanted to.

When he opened his eyes, he was not surprised to see himself lying inside one of Chaudhary's rooms.

"So Chaudhary hangs his gun on that wall!

"The gun has so much dust and cobwebs on it. Fancy Murali being afraid of it."

Ten

Murali had found a treasure. He found it while boarding the train. It was stuck on the footboard of the compartment. Nobody had noticed it. Men all around him looked with indifference while they boarded and got down.

Murali had to wait till the last man got up. Only then he pulled it out. He was expecting someone to come and look for it. So he waited by the door till the train started moving. The purse remained inside his shirt. Safe. Murali knew that he could keep it when even after two stations, no one came looking for it. But he dared not check what was inside it. Why should he make people suspect anything?

"And what could be inside it?"

Murali guessed. Small guesses as well as big guesses. Five rupees guess as well as fifty rupees guess. He continued selling margossa twigs. He continued dreaming around the guesses. He would buy a lottery ticket!

He needed a quiet place to find out what was there inside the purse. "What if there was more than fifty rupees?" Dreams got piled up. Random dreams. Every dream contained the purse which was so close to his skin.

"What was the colour of the purse?

"Was it black or dark brown?"

He could not remember. He walked towards the toilet. Only when he had locked the door did he open the purse. He counted everything. Bills and coins. Twenty-one rupees. Whatever it was, it was a blessing. For he had earned only eight rupees that morning.

He bought himself breakfast for the first time, spending from the black purse, careful not to mix it up with his earned eight rupees. He bought some green marbles for Dasu and coloured beads for Grandmother. He had never seen Grandmother wearing beads, although Murali took for granted that she would not mind keeping some. She should keep them "just like that."

He still had ten rupees left with him. What should he do with it? So he bought some coloured ribbons for their hut. He would hang them around from all the nails of the wall. "Just like that."

Murali came back to the village with his earned eight rupees, glass marbles, coloured beads, coloured ribbons, and a big secret.

Eleven

Dasu had taught his secret to Mustaq. And Mustaq had taught it to Rafiq.

So when every morning, after sitting for ten minutes, somebody or the other started to faint, Chaudhary naturally became suspicious. Anyone would be.

Thus, after five days, when Ali fainted, Chaudhary called his son to tickle the boy to check for himself whether Ali was really sick or not. Poor Ali. He had to stand on one leg for an hour as punishment.

Chaudhary's school had fewer and fewer students with the progress of time. The heaviest blow came to the school when Chaudhary's own son fainted on the tenth day!

And after that, what? Kumar, the teacher, left the village

after that. He got a job in the town as a clerk in a cloth mill after that. Dasu became a full-time cowherd after that. He even began to smell like cows, as grandmother complained, after that. Murali put fewer restrictions on him after that.

And as promised, Dayaram had taken Dasu for a "jail visit." Kirpal was growing a beard for reasons known only to him.

"Who can be this man talking with my father's voice?" Dasu wondered. He would not go near Kirpal. Only when Kirpal showed the pack of cards and shuffled them in front of Dasu was the little boy convinced. For who else could make that purring sound while shuffling cards other than his father?

Dasu was impressed. In fact he was so impressed by Kirpal's beard and his checked prisoner's clothes that he wanted to become a prisoner like Kirpal, then and there. "Do they allow the cows to stay also?"

Dayaram had to fight him to bring him back. The little boy showed every resistance possible. He kicked, he bit and threw tantrums. He however stopped when Dayaram bought him a sweet from a vendor in the train.

The effect of his prison visit stayed with Dasu. He boasted about his father's prison stay to Mustaq and Ali. And he boasted about it so much that everybody wanted to have an experience of a "dream stay" in the prison.

And when Murali started a policeman story, Dasu refused to hear any of it. "Tell me a prisoner story."

Twelve

"Lots and lots of water drops make rain. And all the raindrops come from the distant clouds which live beyond all the seven seas," Grandmother was telling Dasu and Murali while Murali was baking chapatis.

Frogs croaked outside on the puddles made by rain, the sound of which grew louder as the night thickened around their hut. Murali missed the radio which two years back their father had bought from a secondhand shop. Murali remembered how they would listen to it during such rainy nights. And that would turn such a mournful sound of the raindrops more cheerful. And even the croaking frogs seemed to sing with the songs of the transistor radio.

Now with the transistor radio sold and father in the lockup, Murali found the rainy evening very incomplete. Murali missed Kirpal very much. As if it was his father who lived beyond the seven seas. He remembered how Kirpal would come happily back from Giridhari's wine shop and play the transistor while they had their supper. Giridhari had met him this evening to find out how Kirpal was doing in the prison.

Perhaps the rains missed Kirpal too. Shadows on the wall looked longer. Grandmother's old shadow, Dasu's little shadow, and his own big shadow, because he was closest to the oil lamp — everything looked with long faces at him. A great shadow of their missing father was on everything. The everythings included the big black box where grandmother stored secrets, the mud walls on which hung Dasu's kite and the coloured ribbons which Murali had once bought "just like that" after finding a purse in a train, the rope cots, the piled blankets on them, which smelled of dampness, and all those aluminum cooking and serving pots piled out there.

However the smell of hunger arising from the stomachs covered other things because chapatis smelled inside the spaces which were shadowed with emptiness. Dasu was the first to eat. And as he bit the green chili with his first bite of his chapati, he cheered up.

"And who calls the clouds, Grandmother?"

"Oh, the frogs call them because farmers pray to the frogs." Grandmother yawned.

"And why do frogs croak when rains pour, Grandmother?" Dasu wanted to learn more.

"Because they tell all those farmers that their prayers have been answered."

The rains poured, each drop continued to tell its own story, which got included in some greater story.

Thirteen

They had all gone there. Hari, Ratan, Bhoj Singh, Rahim and Soora. Others came after that. Rafiq and his father came when they heard of it from Bhoj Singh. Ratan told Chaudhary's bodyguards. And all the others told each other.

Women came too. But they stood at a distance from the men with curious looks.

The man sat on Dayal's doorway with a bowl of puffed rice and chili talking to Dayal's wife.

"Dayal's brother-in-law," Hari whispered to Ratan. And Ratan whispered it to Rafiq's father.

"Very big man!" Mustaq's father told Rahim. And Rahim told the others.

A guest in the village. Everyone waited to be introduced. The men looked at Dayal, while the women looked at his wife.

Dayal was fanning his brother-in-law. He pretended not to notice anyone. Gopal's mother waved at Dayal's wife, hoping to be introduced first. Dayal's wife did not wave back.

Dasu was there too. Since Murali had gone to the town and grandmother was too weak to come, he thought that he should represent them and show his face to Dayal's brother-in-law. Of course he had brought the two cows with him. For he could not let them graze on their own. Rafiq and Mustaq had also brought their goats along with them. Everyone presented themselves in front of the visitor.

"And he has come all the way from Delhi where the prime minister lives," Mustaq whispered.

"Did you see his umbrella?"

"And did you see his shoes?"

While Dasu was trying to look at the shoes and the umbrella, the white cow of Dayaram somehow entered Dayal's garden and started feeding on his jasmine bush. The black cow followed faithfully. Dasu followed them to chase them out. But the cows embarrassed him because of their disobedience in front of the guest who had come from Delhi where the prime minister stayed.

Dayal cursed everyone and ran out to chase all the three — beasts and boy — out. He picked up the visitor's umbrella in a hurry because there was no stick around to punish them.

Dasu retained the mark which the umbrella had made on his back for a couple of days. Everyone had left after that. They took Dasu along with them. The visitor had left before evening, leaving the umbrella behind. Dayal uses it when he walks across the fields.

Dayal's wife is not called anymore to participate in the women's afternoon gossip-meetings.

Fourteen

Kirpal had returned back from the prison with a long beard. He came back one evening when Dasu had already fallen asleep and Grandmother was counting the coins which Murali had earned.

Money was never enough. And enough had no limits.

A meal which was enough for them left them with something which was not enough. Whenever it rained, the roof started leaking. It needed enough straw to cover it. Murali needed an umbrella to cover his head when he left on those pouring mornings. The plastic sheet which he had been using now to cover his head was not enough. Grandmother tried to count and recount as the vacant spaces of "not enough" stared back at her. Murali and she sat side by side by the oil lamp, trying to fill the spaces of "not enoughs" as best as they could.

Rains had stopped, but the toads continued to croak with the loudest possible croaks all around the hut. And then through the uncertainty of those spaces, Kirpal pushed the door and came in. His beard hung around his chin.

The night remained sleepless around them. There was so much to talk. And every talk tried to fill up those empty spaces of "not enoughs" with hopes and dreams.

Kirpal certainly would not sell margossa twigs anymore, as Murali was already doing it. He would be a fortune-teller.

"That will go well with the beard." All he needed was a pair of glasses and a lens. And since he was not sure how much that would cost, he kept all the coins, which grandmother had kept aside for the roof. The man of the house was back to decide which emptiness to fill first.

Was the night too long? Murali was glad when he heard the first crow of the morning. For all those empty spaces of "not enoughs" got filled with the morning light. He had to start right away. For the seven o'clock local train would not wait for him. But he finished cleaning and washing before leaving.

Dasu was terribly upset when he found his father back. Now how will he visit the prison? He had promised his friends that he would take them all next time!

The sun came out. It dried up the water and tears.

Fifteen

Kirpal came home happy and drunk. He was singing a popular song, which was nothing unusual of him. Murali was expecting him to fall asleep and snore out his breaths.

But tonight, Kirpal sat down in front of Grandmother. He took things out from a bag which looked new to Murali. He wore a pair of thick framed glasses which he had bought from a drama company, and placed a book of palmistry in front of him. An old tattered book. "How do I look?" he asked Murali with a wink.

"When did he learn how to read?" Murali wondered. Kirpal guessed it and winked at him again. Only Grandmother looked concerned. "If the police catch you again?" She sounded alarmed. Kirpal was not worried. "Nobody starves in a prison."

And what if he did go there again? He would just change his trade. There are lots of trades in this world. All you need is to try your hands at everything that you can do. That's all. And life is too short for you to try out those everythings.

Murali served him the last of the chapatis. The night closed around them as the oil of the lantern got over. And deeper breaths of sleep could be heard around. But nobody could hear any of that. For each of their tired ears heard their dreams which each of their tired eyes showed.

Murali dreamt of Chaudhary's goat. He could not tell why he dreamt of it. Chaudhary's goat, in his dream, was reading the same book on palmistry which his father had bought from the town. "When did he learn how to read?" Murali thought in his dream. Perhaps the goat guessed it. It winked at him.

Kirpal saw his own dream while Murali continued dreaming his. Kirpal dreamt of those glasses which he got from a drama company. And it was only through that dream

Kirpal came to know that the glasses could read even if the eyes wearing them could not. The problem arose only when those glasses refused to tell the eyes what they were reading.

Dasu dreamt of the prison castle where he lived with Dayaram's cows. Dayaram's black cow and white cow. The prison castle had many jasmine bushes for the cows to feed on. And in the prison castle, he allowed visitors. Mustaq and Rafiq could come in with their goats. And Dayaram's wife could come in with coconut curry.

Grandmother too must have dreamt of something. Maybe of a new roof with new hay which did not leak when rains poured.

Sixteen

However, rains poured and rains stopped. There was no new hay on the roof. And after a while, the leaking roof began to get unnoticed. Drops of water became a trickle. And Grandmother placed a pot under that, to prevent the water from flowing inside the floor of the hut. And everything got used to each other.

Everyone got used to Kirpal's beard. And Kirpal got used to going to town and telling fortunes by reading the palms of people.

"Why, sir, you shall win the elections some day." Kirpal forced the fruit seller's palm to be placed under his lens. The fruit seller had sat under the same tree in the midday heat.

The fruit seller blushed with a little hope and a little disbelief. And then with a greater hope and lesser disbelief came near Kirpal. He could not pay him with rupees. He could pay him bananas worth the palm reading. By the end of the palm reading, Kirpal had taught the poor man how to dream rich. "And when you become the minister and go to Delhi, remember this fortune teller!"

The fruit seller wanted to know how soon it should happen. Kirpal made heavy calculations. "Fifteen years from the next new moon," Kirpal certified. But he needed to see the position of the stars before telling anything. "I shall become old." The poor man sounded disappointed. The fruit seller wished to see the "tomorrow" today. Kirpal blessed the man. "Dream through your life. And live for your dream."

The fruit seller brought a cobbler with him the next day. And the cobbler brought the flower seller. Kirpal became very busy as palms started to force themselves under his lens.

Grandmother's empty hands began to save once again as dreams began to be sold in the town. Sometimes on this road and sometimes on that road. Sometimes behind the old mosque and sometimes on the railway platform.

Murali heard the sound of a radio once again. For Kirpal had bought a new transistor radio with all the savings. "The roof can wait for a time being for the new hay. But isn't it important to hear the music on a pouring evening?"

The leaking roof waited after hearing the argument.

And everyone got used to the pouring evenings hearing the loud songs from the transistor radio, sitting around it. The leaking roof, too, got used to all of that.

For Grandmother had started saving once again.

Seventeen

The moon was shining in the quietness of the late evening. The rainy season was gone, and Murali's village awaited the winter. Snakes had not yet gone for hibernation and leeches formed colonies everywhere.

However, Grandmother was relieved. For the roof had stopped leaking. And perhaps the moon on the sky was relieved because it became the queen of the night once again.

But tonight Grandmother was worried.

Murali carried a flashlight while he walked across the mustard field. He wished his flashlight could glow brighter when he was walking past the pond where Dulal's wife had drowned herself last winter when Dulal had brought a second wife. Murali walked through Chaudhary's guava plantations, across the barren field where the people have seen strange things and avoid during the new moon nights. Murali was walking towards the railway station.

At home Grandmother was worried. Who else could be more worried other than Murali and Grandmother, when Kirpal had not returned yet from the town? There was, however, the last train to arrive. The twelve o'clock train by which Dinu the beggar usually comes back to the village.

Grandmother was worried. Murali had decided to come to the railway station and wait for his father. Grandmother and Dasu would stay at home. At least Murali could get some news of Kirpal from Dinu the beggar.

Murali hummed a tune to chase the evil spirits off. Dinu had seen them grazing in the darkness. Dinu had told him once how they make horrible faces at you if they see that you are afraid of them. Dinu sings. Dinu sings because spirits are afraid of songs. Murali sang too. He looked around to make sure that the ghost which had its feet bound towards its backward direction was not following him.

"And be careful of leeches," Grandmother had warned him. "They can suck every drop of your blood, leaving you dry."

Murali walked with his worries, fear, and his flashlight. He left every leech and every ghost behind him.

Eighteen

The lights of the signals showed that the railway station was nearby. He had the last hurdle to cross. The wasteland where nobody farmed anything because nothing would grow. Dinu knew everything about it. Why shouldn't he know? Wasn't he the oldest man in the village? "Nothing grows there because it is the grazing ground of the strange horse whose rider has no head," Dinu told him. "But they can only be seen on new moon nights."

Murali looked up at the moon. The strange horse should not come under the moon. But who knows? He ran across the wasteland and stopped only when he had reached the station.

The gypsies were sitting around a fire singing some cheerful tune in some unknown language. Murali sat at a distance and watched them sing. He wished to become a gypsy, sleeping under a silver moon. The gypsies ignored him completely. Murali could not see the monkey anywhere. "Where do they keep the animals?"

And then Murali remembered that he was worried. And back home Grandmother was worried. Dasu was concerned too. His father had promised to bring a parrot for him from the town. The train arrived with a loud roar. Dinu got down. And behind him was Kirpal. Kirpal was limping as Murali ran towards them. He held Dinu's shoulders while Dinu limped on his walking stick. Murali had not seen his father in so much pain before.

Questions came and went in his mind. "What could have happened?" came in every form before Murali.

They brought him back home. Dinu and Murali. Dinu helped as much as his old bones could do.

Kirpal was badly hurt. He could tell nothing that night. All the questions remained around him with dumb expectations waiting for the day. Kirpal groaned with pain. The only answer he could give that night.

Nineteen

Kirpal was badly beaten up that day.

How could Kirpal guess that the man whom he had told about his son's getting a job soon would find him out and seek an explanation from him because his son did not get the job? And how could Kirpal know that the frustrated man would get him beaten up?

"His face is badly swollen," Dayaram observed.

Grandmother kept a cloth pad dipped in warm water on Kirpal's cheekbone. It had turned blue.

Murali left for the seven o'clock train. He needed to continue selling the margossa twigs to keep the kitchen fire burning.

And he knew that the kitchen fire now depended on him. At least till Kirpal got well enough to pursue some wild dream.

Dasu had left too with the cows. He knew that he had to wait for his parrot for some time.

Kirpal soothed his pain with a new dream. He would start a shop like Dayaram. The shop would grow big. He would ask Murali to help him out when the shop grew big. Then the shop would grow bigger. He would need Dasu to help him out when the shop grew bigger.

Slowly, when everything would look small compared to the shop, he would sell it. He would sell it because he would get bored with it. The shop would open its door and look at him with a boring yawn.

But who would he sell the shop to? He would certainly not sell the shop to Chaudhary. Even if Chaudhary pleaded. How could he sell it to such a big man? He would sell it to the gypsies who have camped at the railway platform. In exchange, he would take their camp.

The rest of it was a "gypsy dream." Then with some pain and some fever, Kirpal sold all those dreams to himself.

While Grandmother bought all those worries. She paid a teardrop for them.

Murali sold margossa twigs to passengers.

Dasu did not sell anything at all. He bought every drop of sunbeam from the sky under which Dayaram's cows grazed. He paid for them. He paid for them with his childhood.

Grey, Apple Green, and White

Salvador Dalí paints his dreams, and I write my dreams. This piece is a tribute to my favorite painter.

Grey

Just when the clouds began to settle down on the hills, just when the sun became tired of shining and shining and decided to take a little rest behind those clouds, and just when the wind began to grow noisy, the earth seemed to vanish between the colours of grey and more grey.

All around was grey. The leafless tree standing all alone waiting for spring to be covered with leaves again looked grey. The grass that was left around to grow on the little soil clinging to those rocks looked grey. I suppose the wind had a colour too. It was grey.

His little body, covered with hunger and dust, descended slowly down the narrow road through the wind and through the grey.

And the little dog that had been following him ever since he left the outskirts of the previous city looked a darker grey.

The animal kept a little distance from his footsteps, not yet sure whether it would be proper to walk closer.

He did not notice anything. Not even those clouds, which could begin to bring rain any moment. Not even those lumps of rocks lying around waiting for something to happen. He did not wait. How could he wait when there was his dream right on the lids of his eyes, making him see nothing else but its sunshine colours of orange and purple and green?

The silver moonlight had once whispered about that dream, in his ears.

And where should he find that dream?

It was right around somewhere, the silver moonlight had promised him. All he needed to do was look carefully around him.

Ever since, he has been looking for nothing but his dream. So how could he see the clouds, the rocks, or the little dog, which was following him? It was hungry and tired like him.

Both of them were coloured in grey.

Apple Green

Maybe it was a little stir on those leaves. Perhaps a little bird just flew off from a slender branch. Maybe a little air pushed off just to let him know that it was time to move on.

The dog got up.

So did he.

A few moments passed by while he gathered his bag and hung it on his shoulder. It did not matter anyway what was there inside it. Perhaps there was his spare shirt and spare slippers. Was his flute there too? He tried to feel the flute and found it there.

Would that dog listen if he played it here?

He had to sit. And he had to play the "apple green" tune. The tune could colour the world with apple green. In this wild land, what else could colour the world better, if not apple green?

He began. Who knows what the dog thought about it? But it sat down right next to him.

The leaves stirred around. The thin branches moved. And green and brown started getting mixed up into one colour.

Apple green.

The earth and wind began to breathe in apple green. They surely loved the sound of apple green.

✻   ✻   ✻

The dog was the last to be coloured with apple green. It moved its head so much that the colour would not settle easily. Its brown and white body would curl up and now and then would stir up with slightest sound caused by the leaves. But it heard all of the tune. Only when all the apple green settled on its ears, eyes, and paws did he stop playing.

He was hungry. He got up. He had to find food for himself and the dog. Then he had to continue looking for his dream. His sunshine-coloured dream, of orange and purple and green, just as the silver moonlight had promised him.

The dog got up too.

They were leaving the boundaries of apple green.

White

They said it was white.

Some said for sure it was whiter than those clouds, which were writing some sort of a script on the wide space of the sky.

What were those clouds writing anyway? He wanted to know. Did the dog care about it?

He had to wait for it now and then because the animal had tiny legs and was getting tired every "once in a while." He did not mind waiting. It gave him time to watch those clouds cover the sky with "who knows what" script.

"It is white for sure," one of them said.

"You will not miss the tall dome," the other said.

"Anyone can see it from a distance."

"And everyone is allowed in."

He waited for the dog once again. It had spotted a yellow and black butterfly.

He continued hearing from them. They continued telling.

"And you do not need to worry about entering there. There are no doors that open or close. And there are no guards who let you in or stop you."

"You do not need to seek any place there. For everyone has a place."

The dog chased the yellow and black butterfly around. And the clouds were still halfway through the sky. "Wonder what they wrote till now.

"Perhaps they were writing a whole story of a butterfly.

"A yellow and black butterfly."

The dog, however, lost sight of the insect and returned to him. He turned where their fingers pointed so that he could reach it while there was still daylight. He needed to be patient.

The dog spotted it first. He allowed the animal to lead the way.

The animal hesitated. It is easy for an animal to trust

human beings, but never easy for it to trust the house of prayer. And why should there be reason for it to trust a house of prayer anyway? It is not expected to be seen inside it.

The dog slowed down.

"All are welcomed there." He understood the animal's hesitation.

They entered. Both human and beast were covered in white light, which filtered through the white dome. No door opened and no door closed.

There was no door. There was no boundary. Every prayer had the same colour: white.

And every dream had the same colour: white.

For every colour of the sunshine, orange or purple or green, when they joined hands, merged into one colour, white.

He saw his dream in the colour of his prayer. It was all around him. It belonged to everyone who was there around him, including the dog. It did not matter whether anyone had come in search of any dream or not. The universal dream belonged to all.

He got up after the dog. He needed to turn back and find his way home through the colours of apple green and grey. There was no need for him to travel for his dream. He looked up at the sky.

The clouds had filled the sky. They completed writing a prayer in the sky.

Impressive People

People are always interesting. People are always impressive. This piece is my humble tribute towards some impressive people I met somewhere in my experience of life.

One

There are many kinds of people around us. Some sure are more impressive than others. An impressive person carries his expressions masked with a kind of crude indifference. He walks the streets, sits on the backseats of a bus, and watches the world as it turns from morning to noon. And he tries to avoid any form of eye contact with anyone, although you can be very sure that he is watching you with some gifted vision of his.

You try to show off your friendly gesture by opening the first page of a recently bought magazine to tempt him to at least look at you.

No, he is just not bothered by the reason for the bankruptcy of Enron which is discussed on the open page.

Then you try to flutter the pages right in front of his eyes so that the green and orange and blue colours of the glossy pages shine his face up. Yet his eyes do not turn.

Next you try to flutter it right in front of his face to air his nose. At least he would breathe out the irritation.

He sits like a rock.

And he waits. He waits for your next attention-seeking approach.

And you give up. No, not quite. You tickle your nostril with the corner of your facial tissue and sneeze.

It works, finally. He tries to breathe out harder and harder, so that the last speck of bacteria is chased out.

You see the pages of your magazine flutter, although there is no wind blowing. But you know why. He is breathing out bacteria on the pages.

Two

Impressive people can be found in a shopping mall.

They can really impress anyone by the amount of reading they do to gain knowledge. They usually pick up a product and hold it higher than their eye level before starting to actually read the different ingredients and instructions for using the product.

And certainly they become voracious readers when they realise that you are around them with your curious eyes turning into that look of admiration.

They read and you watch.

They read and you get curious.

They read and you look inside your shopping basket at all those items you have collected without even reading anything. All those "everythings" with those labels printed there for your eyes to see.

Surely you could have learnt something about the ingredients. The product may contain fifty grams of sodium meta bisulphate or twenty-nine grams of calcium bicarbonate. And that may be one or two grams less than what you actually need.

So you try to stay close to your inspiration and pick up a packet to show everyone that you are as product-literate as anyone.

You pick up the product to the same height above your eye level, to get a proper light and the right amount of inspiration. You read and try to understand everything about the twenty percent sodium phosphate which the product contains. Would twenty grams be better than twenty-five grams? Take an average? How fast can you calculate?

Then you wonder whether you should go for the one which has 22.9 percent sodium hydrogen phosphate. Since then, you try to stay close to the people who have impressed you. Who knows how many more things they will teach you?

Sure enough, shopping will be a learning experience for you next time.

Three

Impressive people can be found anywhere. In fact, you need not even have to go around looking for them.

You look around you, and there he stands in the corner with his face buried in the pages of a thick book.

Shame on every other person, who cannot even read on a busy bus-stop bench. Fools do not even know that there is so much to read and so little time. And so short a life. You try to look inside your bag to find something worth reading. Maybe you had kept something, which must have been there since then, waiting for the right moment to come.

But all your hands dig out is a two-month-old receipt.

Next time you need to be more careful. Perhaps carry a bigger bag so that it can hold at least a paperback.

Your bus comes and you are relieved. At least you do not have to bother anymore about your time being wasted.

The impressive person gets up just behind you and chooses to sit, out of all those places in the bus, right next to you.

And he opens to page number 999 of the *Best Speeches of the Twentieth Century*.

You try to look away but you cannot. You cannot, because you are attracted by the example of "devoted concentration" sitting right next to you.

Will you try to distract him?

Yes, you may try. So you try to change your sitting position, and you give him an elbow nudge.

He just ignores you and turns the page.

Next, you try to drop your bag right at his feet and bend all your weight down to pick it up, not forgetting to say a "sorry."

The eyes roll a bit. The feet move a bit, and the page turns once more.

But now your stop has come and you have to get down.

So with an "Excuse me," you try to come out of your seat. You leave him and his *Best Speeches of the Twentieth Century* there in the bus.

Every one has his destiny.

And everyone has so much to learn.

Four

I have tried to draw my inspiration from a friend of my brother's friend's husband's nephew, whom I met a few months ago when I heard him talk.

It was at a social function.

And it happened to be that all of us were present there. My brother, his friend, her husband, and his nephew.

✻   ✻   ✻

It so happened that all of us gathered there as if to realise the remarkable potential which this young man was carrying. He had gathered a pretty reasonable group of admirers around him, which made me get inquisitive at first.

My first motive was just to peep in and not get too involved with the "whatever-that-was-going-on."

And then I heard terms like hydrogen concentration of hemispheric haemoglobin causing the hypercromosomic anaemia.

And then I heard of neuroplasmatic effect on the newly formed neurons causing imbalance of nephroreorganisation.

"Wow."

And that was the beginning. I never realised that a simple human body could have such technical functions, with all those different kinds of remarkable activities. The crowd grew around that evolving area of information and knowledge. I wondered whether I had had one of those geohydrolic effects of gastrointestinal pressure when I burped in the middle of a pleasant conversation with the young lady I just met at the gathering a while ago, which left me all embarrassed.

How long did I stay there gathering information and admiring those complicated terms? I have no idea. But it was a while, long enough to leave me stranded outside because the last bus had gone. I was however rescued by a drunk stranger who wanted to do his last good deed for the day by giving me a ride.

And how could I refuse when both of us were in need of each other?

And the ride is another story of inspiration by itself.

Five

He was standing on the steps of the public library. He carried some books in his hands.

Very thoughtful.

The world was moving around him while he was moving around his thoughts. People climbed up the steps and down the steps all around him. He did not notice anyone.

A discoverer of a certain law of nature. Or an inventor of a complicated logical imbalance theory. "What mathematical factor determines the miseries of mankind?"

I watched him with keen interest and admiration. I had never seen a live inventor or discoverer before. And I did not want to miss my opportunity to watch him. What was he watching from behind those heavy glasses?

I saw all those heavy books he was holding. Heavy old books. History? Civilisation? Inorganic chemistry? Or maybe mathematics.

A thinker of the present century.

When the world has grown too busy to think, here was a perfect example of one of the few representatives of the human race who still spend time thinking.

I could imagine all those galaxies he was looking at by merely turning his eyes on the road. I could imagine all those blue dreams he was looking at by merely turning towards the blue sky. And I could imagine all those mathematical equations getting solved in his mind as he looked at the countless stream of people around him.

I had to go.

I walked across the street and turned back to have a last look at him.

He stood there with his books and with his thoughts.

Very impressive.

Six

He sat right in front of me in the airport lounge. He wore a black tie which hung around his neck like a big embrace of importance. And sure he went out to seek something important.

I could tell that from his impatient eyebrows. And I could tell it from his brown briefcase, which I was sure contained every kind of important this and that. I waited for it to get opened, and it soon did.

Papers, files, and all kinds of letters were seen peeping out and rushing out as he tried to take something out and then took out something else by mistake and tried it again. He was the most important man in the lounge, I observed. A well-deserved "important man of the day."

I shrunk to my place, not daring to move to disturb his thoughts and his watch, which he consulted time and again.

And time and again, he tried to call some number and got frustrated. "Who-was-he" who could not answer his very important call? It made me share some of his impatience too. He took out some papers from his case. Went through them very carefully and put them back again. Then he remembered something which he had forgotten to read and took those papers out once more. And allowed the cycle to be repeated again. Then once again.

I needed to sit close to him so that I could get a proper look at him and get the right kind of motivation to move in life. What was a life, after all, that did not even have any motivation? So when a gentleman who was sitting next to him got up because he was not getting any kind of inspiration from all that movement, I took his place. Very important lines from one paper got very carefully read. But every time I tried to peep into those papers, he kept them back, not wanting to share the important secrets.

I did not give up. I needed the kind of motivation in life where I could feel the importance of papers and time too. So he had no right to ignore me.

I asked him the time. He looked at my wrist where my watch faced us both. And he read aloud the time by consulting my watch, making me feel very embarrassed.

And then I suppose he got uncomfortable because of my presence. Otherwise, why should he look at me with that unfriendly and suspicious frown?

I saw him get up, collecting all those papers. I saw him pack up his briefcase and leave the place.

Very impressive.

Impressive people need not always be friendly.

Little Grains of Dust

I love gypsies. I wish I could own nothing, not even my name, just like those little grains of dust. They inspired me to write this piece.

Little Beginning

> Little heart aches and a little pain
> Little sorrow and a little gain
> Little of sun and little of rain
> With little to go and little to gain.
> A little to hear and a little to say
> A little to take and a little to pay
> A little of rest under a little shade
> To seek the dust grains on the way.

Little dust grains could be seen all around me. Little dust grains scattered in the air, floating with their own sublime peace, little dust grains with the wheels of the trucks suddenly breaking their peace and flying with a wakeful alertness, little dust grains in my breaths and of course little dust grains on and around the road, making a greater togetherness to form a dusty everything. Dusty road, dusty air, dusty bushes around the road, dusty fields, and of course a dusty self of mine with my dusty feet.

And the road ahead of me had a little of everything.

There was a little of road and a little of cracks. It had a little of sun and a little of shade. It was a little narrow here and a little broad there. There was a little speed and a little rest. And above all there was a little of hope and a little of memories which were all along with me while I walked.

I had walked on the road with the little steps of mine to cover a long distance. There was no hurry. I did not bother about my destiny because I did not have one. However I was sure that the road was leading me to Somewhere. The Somewhere could be anywhere on the earth. It could be any city or any village or any place which was not a big city and not any village either. And sure, I was a little tired. But I walked and continued to walk till all those little tirednesses grouped and joined together into a greater tiredness and made me stop.

I waited for a greater end to my little footsteps. Dusty footsteps.

Greater End

And greater end it did come
When the road took me

Through a place which was none
Other than my new destiny.

The greater end came when I saw the smoke-filled horizon. It grew at first into an outline of tall chimneys, which became distinct and showed the broad chimneys of a factory. Steel factory.

And there was a fresh hope entering my mind. But my hope was not as high as the tall chimneys. "Sure, I can find some job there."

And then what else? I made my new stay in the new place within its definiteness. And the definiteness was none other than the door number 13, in Refugee Colony of Ashoknagar.

Ashoknagar. Where the new steel factory had brought in people like me. People whose hopes were not as high as the tall chimneys of the steel factory where they worked. Hopes remained touching the ground, where there was still a lot of dust.

My house was a tin-and-plastic-made shelter with a tin sheet door. Although I did not need a door because there was nothing worth taking from my shelter. However every shelter needed a door in the Refugee Colony because the door needed a number. The door number was needed by the owner of the Refugee Colony whenever he came to collect the rent.

So I had a door and my door had a number. I, who did not even have a proper name, had a door. Fancy door!

I needed a name in Ashoknagar as I needed it elsewhere, in Bhawanipur or in Jhumripur. So I called myself Mukund here in Ashoknagar, as I called myself Shamlal in Bhawanipur and Rahamatullah in Jhumripur. Of course there were other names and places also.

The main advantage of not having any name sticking to you is this. You can call yourself anything. When you get bored of people calling you Habib, you can immediately leave the place and call yourself Mukund. The world is too vast to stay, and names are plenty to keep. As plenty as the grains of dust.

It was easy to find a shelter, as nobody wanted to live in unlucky 13, although the owner charged less for it. I had no problem.

> And so for the time of the next
> I shall dwell in the new found place
> And my name shall be the same
> Until I am tired of the very name.

My Name

And the name may be any
Yet myself will call it "me"
For the heart which makes the beat
Beats the same in wake or sleep.

My shadow that has followed me even here reminds me of all those names by which I was known. So sometimes I forget that I am Mukund of Ashoknagar who sells tea outside the factory gate. It reminds me that I was Shamlal the thief of Bhawanipur. It reminds me that I was Habib the house servant when I was in Shantigarh, and it also reminds me that it was the same shadow of Rabu the gypsy.

My thoughts get interrupted by the factory siren because it is the time of my business for the day. Workers come one by one out of the gate. Some of them go to Banwari's betel shop, some of them go to the Favourite Tea Stall, while others come to me. They know that I shall be ready with my kettle and plastic tumblers. They know that my special tea costs much less than what the owner of the Favourite Tea Stall charges. And everyone knows that my special tea has more sugar compared to what the shop offers.

I run from one corner to another under the shade of the margossa tree, calling out to those tired, furnace-burnt faces, inviting one and all to have my tea.

I am not really worried about setting up a shop like the Favourite Tea Stall, although I can if I want. Stability is too much of a burden for me. Having a definite name and place and seeing the shadow within the domain of that definiteness is too much of a load.

I do not allow any stability for me.

In the prison while I stayed there for three months the law-keepers had asked me all those questions which any name holder should have.

When I told them the truth about my names and dwellings they did not believe me. So I had to call myself a different name in the prison. The police recorded me as Motia, village Sankurria.

When my stay of three months got over, I stopped calling myself Motia. Since I was a petty thief and a pickpocket, I was released earlier than all my other prison mates.

"Where will you go?" I was asked.

"To my village at Sankurria," I had assured them. "I will till the farm and look after my ailing father."

I had left the place then and there because my companions knew me as Shamlal while the police knew me as Motia of village Sankurria. My shadow had followed.

My Shadow

> And my shadow
> Made a follow
> No matter where I went
> Walking my steps
> Waiting my rests
> All the long distance

The time was three P.M., and the workers came out of the factory gate once again for the afternoon tea break. There was no time at all to look at my shadow that time. For it was time to follow Munna bhai, Rajam Rao, Kishenlal, Mohammed Hussain, and all of them who were thirsty for tea. My shadow followed me.

My shadow had also followed me on all those times when I had nothing to follow in particular, on all those times when I had the blankness of chasing nothing. I chased all those nothingness of the unknown anythings, it could be a butterfly on a mustard cultivation, yellow as the mustard flowers. It could be a floating eagle or it could be the white cloud which had suddenly appeared from behind some distant horizon. It could be chasing even some dust grains which flew in a nowhere direction. I, chasing those anythings, and my shadow chasing me.

The afternoon was too bright for people to stay in the hot sun. Most of them had collected under the big margossa tree, under which, last month, some of them had gone for an indefinite hunger strike. Mohammed Hussain, Motilal, Kishenlal, Sukhia, and others were there. Their dusty hair and unshaven faces showed their great determination.

It was during that time I had found that they were chasing some cause. I stayed with them with my own inquisitiveness because I had to find out how it felt like when you chased a cause. I felt a kind of brotherhood with them as the days of their strike progressed. However, I never even bothered to find out what they were demanding.

I never had to be in a position which needed any demand. For demands grow from responsibility. And I have not faced any so far. I don't even own a name to be responsible for. And my shadow is too mute to demand anything from me.

> The strike had ended anyway
> As do end all things
> But I had learnt how men say
> About their demanding.
> And I had shared, but for once
> The same roof under the skies
> With those men who drank my tea
> Under it otherwise.

Heart Throbs

> Heart can throb in many ways
> Fast or slow may be
> The beats are yet inside the self
> My eye does never see.

Heart throbs occur within me whenever Manju passes by my door number 13. I try to turn my eyes away, elsewhere, because they are the root of all my heart throbs. I usually look away towards the ugliest part of my room behind my door. A hole at the back tin wall through which the smoke enters in the mornings and through which the smell of the drain enters during those damp summer evenings. Beauty is thus humiliated by the ugliness.

However heart throbs continue as my eyes see the hole, while my mind continues to see Manju crossing the road and then going to the rickshaw stand where Motilal would be waiting for her.

I continue to see the hole as I continue to think about Manju. Manju talking to Motilal. Manju giggling at something funny she had just heard. Manju talking this and Manju talking that. The rickshaw stand and Manju. The setting sun of the evening behind the park which is behind the rickshaw stand and behind which is Manju.

And time passes with me staring at the hole. I open my door number 13 once again to see all those beautiful things beyond it. And heart throbs become beautiful once again.

> I let it throb, fast or slow,
> In whatever way it seeked.
> And my heart judged the best,
> How it would beat.
> Whatever the reason be
> My heart throbbed its way
> For those which my eyes could see
> I never could hush them away.

The sun continued to set behind Manju, behind Motilal behind the rickshaw stand, behind the park and behind the earth.

My heart continued to throb.

Shamlal

> In the hours when darkness dwells
> And the evils thrive and swell
> The hours pass by in some spell
> In the darkness of my shell

I called him "Ustad the teacher." He called me "Shamlal my pupil."

I had learnt the art of pickpocketing from him. I consider it to be an art because it needed a lot of patience and practice to master it. I was good at it from the very beginning, even better than Babulal, who learnt it from the Ustad the teacher at the same time as me.

Ustad had taught us many things. He taught us how to escape the clutches of a man by removing the shirts from our bodies if he caught a corner of our shirt. He taught us to keep some dust grains with us so that we could sprinkle it into the eyes of anybody who tried to catch hold of us.

Ustad the teacher had come with us to the railway booking counter on our first day at it. He was keeping an eye on our abilities. Since I was better at it, Babulal had to assist me in my job.

"Choose the correct man," Ustad would say. "The correct man's pocket always contains the correct amount in his wallet."

I was a bit nervous in the beginning. However I closed towards a gentleman with a heavy-looking pocket. Babulal knew what to do. He had started a quarrel with Ustad in the queue. Their quarrel drew a lot of attention, including the gentleman with a heavy pocket. I had to act fast while others paid more heed to the quarrel.

When Ustad and Babulal saw me walking out, they called truce. Ustad came out five minutes after Babulal. I was waiting behind the bridge. Only the money was taken from the wallet. The rest, paper and wallet, were thrown into the river. Ustad had rewarded us well. I could even buy Babulal's sister those red bangles which she wanted so much.

I could even confidently carry on the work without the presence of Ustad, because he had to retire for a few weeks after he had broken his leg by falling down from a drainpipe. He had taken us, one night, out on a stealing expedition.

I had been Shamlal for five years. And then one day I was caught while stealing copper wires from an electricity pole. Babulal had fled. I knew then and there that I would leave the town after my release from the jail.

> And then again
> With a new name
> My morning began afresh,
> When on some date
> Out of the prison gate
> I took my road ahead.

They

> They laugh and share
> Their worries and cares
> Under the margossa tree
> While they fill their
> Lungs with air
> Which comes from the tall chimneys

Surkhiram was celebrating the birth of his daughter by treating everybody with betel leaf and tea. He had also distributed a few packets of salted biscuits amongst his friends. He promised to celebrate it in a bigger way next time, when a son would be born. I had to make my "special tea" with a few cloves and cardamoms boiled together with tea leaves and milk.

Orders like this come rarely. However I am always prepared for it. Otherwise the Favourite Tea Stall would grab the offer. And everyone knows that "special tea" costs three rupees a cup.

The men were discussing the birth of the daughter, because Surkhiram had to start saving for her marriage from now. The time of the birth was also important, because the child born on the new moon night was supposed to bring luck to her father. Who knows, Surkhiram could even win the next lottery!

Surkhiram blushed under the shade of the margossa tree and ordered one more kettle of "double special tea," which needed more milk and sugar. I began to prepare the tea while calculating my profit for the day. For everybody knew that "double special tea" would cost four rupees a cup.

I knew exactly what to do with the profit. I would buy a pair of earrings for Manju. The ones which I had seen last week displayed in a glass casing of a travelling seller. The man had told me the price and he would not go below it, even if I offered him tea for free. The red glass beads of the earrings would suit none other but Manju.

☆　　☆　　☆

Tea time was over. Men were going back inside the factory congratulating Surkhiram, predicting all those good fortunes which awaited him and blessing the baby with a good husband when she grows up one day.

As I cleaned up the place which had been blessed with the goodwill and blessings, I wondered about my unknown birth date. Was it also celebrated with special tea and salted biscuits? I knew that my shadow was the only witness of my birth.

For it was also born with me. But it would not tell me anything.

Rahamatullah

The name of the city was as musical as the sound of the bell of my rickshaw. It was Jhumripur. I called myself Rahamatullah. And people called me Rahamatullah the rickshaw puller. My rickshaw had a proper name. I called it the Flying Horse.

Of course I did not own the rickshaw. How could I own anything when I did not even own a name? I had borrowed it from Lakshman Seth, who allowed us to use his rickshaws provided we paid 10 percent of our earnings to him as rent. We were four in number. He had given us a room to stay in his outhouse. My friends were Kantilal, Devilal, and Mahadeo.

> And the peace of each morning
> Heard the bells of our rickshaws ring
> In the hope to start the day
> With the profit from a good earning.

Mahadeo had told us how to be lucky. He told us to keep ringing the rickshaw bells till we found the first passenger for the day. It was lucky. And it was lucky to see the first morning shadow of your rickshaw behind the holy tree where the women came to pray in the mornings.

And who did not wish to get lucky? Even I, Rahamatullah the rickshaw puller, who had no reason whatsoever to get lucky, could not resist the temptation of getting lucky.

The music of our rickshaw bells spread through the streets of Jhumripur along the four directions, east, west, north, and south, as we parted in the four directions at the junction of the holy tree.

> And then the Luck with our selves
> Rang with sureness of our bells
> Morning Luck with growing day
> Started off with a good pay.

Sometimes I met Devilal on the way while I carried passengers from the railway station to the town and he carried passengers from the town to the station. Kantilal's stand was the market, while Mahadeo rang his lucky bell near the temple.

But Luck comes in a bad way also, because it is very whimsical. It came to Mahadeo in its bad way. So one evening after he came back with his rickshaw bell ringing, he found a visitor from his village waiting to see him.

Mahadeo had to go home immediately because his wife had died of cholera. He never returned. I knew that I had to leave Jhumripur.

I had to leave early next morning before Jhumripur woke up and before any shadow appeared on the dust or behind the holy tree. Flying Horse lost its name with me. It has become any other rickshaw with a new rickshaw puller now.

Monkeys on My Roof

The tin-sheet roof of my room is the landing ground for all those monkeys which come down from the jackfruit tree in search of food. In fact, they do not need to search for food, because of Tewari.

Tewari owns a sweet shop at the corner of the Refugee Colony, where the lane links the main road of the market. And Tewari has taken every responsibility to feed every arboreal habitant. "Lord Rama's own beast," explains Tewari.

So he feeds them with all those sweets, free of cost, which he would not give anyone without taking the price.

It is no use telling him that my tin roof is threatened when the monkeys jump on it directly from the jackfruit tree. Tewari would just shake his head at my ignorance. How could I forget that Lord Rama's own beasts act according to Lord's will?

So as soon as the monkey landings start, I come out of my door number 13, along with my kettle and portable oven, and head towards the factory gate under the margossa tree.

Lord Rama's beasts
Hold their feast
Under my tin roof,
So with peace
In the least
I leave the juvenile group.

The monkeys never show any interest in me although I always wave a stick as a precaution. Once Lakhan the fruit seller was surprised by them when one of them had jumped directly from the jackfruit tree on his bananas, before he could even know what was going on. He started carrying a stick like me since then. He even deliberately waves and knocks his stick against the pushcart where he keeps his bananas, only to show those monkeys how prepared he is.

Tewari shakes his head at our fear.

>Monkeys eat and Monkeys play
>All around the place
>Every morning every day
>With the Monkey grace.

I keep waving my stick in the air lest anyone follow.
Lakhan knocks and waves his stick on the banana push-cart. And we walk out of sight.

Dead Ram by My Door

>And the many many days
>When events seem to happen always
>And the always seem parts of time
>And time can be of any kind
>For when the bonds of time do grow
>Into the sureness of events that show
>The age-old earth and moonlit glow
>Is always there like a following shadow.

When the mind knows that things will happen today and tomorrow and the day after, as it happens always, every day, like the rising sun, like the six o'clock factory siren, and like the monkeys landing on my tin roof, the heart takes for granted all of them as a part of every day. And they become so much a part of the day that it becomes very natural to wonder why one of them did not happen if, one morning, another one of them fails to occur.

So when one day the monkeys did not jump on my tin roof, I was naturally worried because the usualness was broken. I came out to find the cause. Was Tewari the monkey feeder unwell? And then I saw the dead ram, Motilal's pet, lying right in front of my door. The monkeys were sitting on the jackfruit tree above me, looking curiously at the dead ram.

"Who brought it here? My monkeys are hungry." Tewari was asking everyone. He was impatient because he was getting late. He opened his shop only after feeding Lord Rama's own beasts. He pleaded with everyone to push the dead beast somewhere called elsewhere, because he had already taken his bath. And everybody knew that after taking his bath, Tewari never touched any dead body. Not even dead rams.

I told him I never touched dead rams too. So did Vinod the cobbler. So did Manju's father Lal Babu. And so did all the others who were amused by the sight of impatient Tewari and the frightened monkeys.

Even Motilal could not be found anywhere. After all, the ram, living or dead, was his pet! The dead ram challenged everyone with its alarming stink as the morning matured.

Finally, Tewari, Lal Babu, and I dragged the dead ram of Motilal somewhere away from the Refugee Colony to save the breaths from the stink. And Motilal came immediately after that to thank us for the service. He touched only living rams.

And after that, the monkeys came down.

Dukhia

> Although I am bothered not
> For any good or bad
> Yet I know that good in man
> Can bring tears from my heart.

I came down with fever once when people knew me as Habib of Kishengunj. It was a rainy season. Dukhia and I shared a small hut when he worked as a domestic servant and I blacked cinema tickets.

The sound of the rain outside our hut, the sound of the croaking frogs, and the sound of the very breaths and coughs of mine became the sound of fever.

And I had wished then that I had a somebody to call my own, like Dukhia had in his village. I had also wished that for once I had a definite name. I thought and I thought in my fever because I had got a lot of nothingness to think about. I wondered whether I had malaria or whether I had typhoid, I calculated the money which was left with me. I surely could not afford any medicine with that.

Dukhia too had to leave for his work early. I was alone with my thoughts, wonders, worries, and wishes around me. The darkness of the hut lay around those thoughts. The rain poured around the hut. And everything was there around the rain. I remained in the centre of the world. And all the everythings remained with their own centres. Maybe all those centres too had their own worries and pains.

> And thus in my fever, sleep or wake
> When the morning was raining wet
> I had wished that I had a name
> And perhaps could be born again.

Dukhia had come back early that day. I could not make out whether it was late morning or whether it was early noon. He had brought some flowers from some temple. Poor man's medicine. He kept them under my pillow, wrapped in a leaf. He put a wet cloth on my forehead and fanned my head.

And thus he became a part of my thoughts, which were a part of my heart. Because it was my heart which was thinking at that time. My thoughts with Dukhia as their part diffused into my sleep to continue into my dreams.

I had got up after three days of wake, sleep, pain, thoughts, and dreams. All that remained after that was only the thoughts which my heart had thought.

I had left the hut with those flowers at night, leaving the money left with me for Dukhia to use. He was sleeping in his own peace, with his own dreams and with his stable name to keep.

I walked away, to seek a new name for me.

Problems

Does the margossa tree know that its leaves are very bitter, and they are taken as medicine? Does it know that we call it the margossa tree? Or does it call itself by some other name? I am sure that it hears Ramdin, Sukhia, and Haribai sit under it and talk about their problems.

Of course all those problems are the common problems of anybody who has a definite name and address. I have never experienced anything like that.

All those problems gather under the shade of the margossa tree and get mixed up with the tea which cooks inside my aluminum kettle. Hot tea, cool shade, and a lot of problems. And some of those problems also get settled on the dusty ground, waiting to fly by any provoking wind.

And Sukhia's problems find consolations in the problems of Ramdin. While Haribai finds consolation of his problems by consoling Sukhia. And they gulp their problem-filled words down with my hot tea.

"Daughter is growing big every day. Yet her marriage cannot be fixed," complains Ramdin. "And I have three more daughters." Ramdin sighs.

"Wife is sick, and medicines are too expensive." Sukhia breathes heavily.

"Why don't you take her to the Pir Baba's tomb?" suggests Haribai.

> And Haribai complains his part.
> Sukhia suggests this and that
> And the tree above hears the talk
> In the stillness around perhaps.

The margossa tree is left alone when they go inside the factory gate after the tea break. No, not quite alone, because I am there too, and there are those grains of dust which get ready to be blown by some stray wind, taking those problems which have settled down on it into some other place.

The margossa tree too must have some secret problems of its own which are mixed up there under it. Maybe those grains of dust settle them too, mixing them with Sukhia's, Haribai's, and Ramdin's problems.

And what about the sky at large,
When I look at it
I doubt the blue sky also has
Some problem there, too, hid.

And while I clean up the place
All those cups and all that mess
I worry nonetheless
For I have problems none to face.

I try hard to find my problem, because I suppose without it there is no purpose in life. But my problem remains some secret question which refuses to be revealed even in my mind. I let it be in that secretness.

Earrings

And again those little things
Make a great beginning
When she smiled a little flash
It seemed like smile unending.

Manju had smiled indeed when she saw the earrings with the red glass bead. She had just smiled. She had said nothing. I had expected nothing more. In fact I had expected nothing at all. I never expect anything because the reactions can be of any kind. Manju could have rejected it, or Manju could have given it away to her sister. And expectations can grow and grow. Sometimes they can grow beyond your control, without your awareness, bigger than you, away from the dusty parts around you, lifting you up to such a height that it really hurts when you have a fall.

And so the flash of her smile was a big gift from her to me. It would give me something to reflect on when I stare at the hole in my room through which the smoke enters during the mornings and through which the smell of the drain enters during those damp evenings.

Her smile was not unfamiliar to me.

When I was Shamlal the thief, when I had bought those red glass bangles for Babulal's sister, I had seen the same sort of smile.

When I was Habib the seller of black cinema tickets, when I had shared the hut with Dukhia the domestic servant, when I had bought Razzia the red scarf, I had seen the same sort of smile.

And when I was Rabu the gypsy, and when I had given Rabbia the trinkets to hang around her waist, I had seen the same sort of smile.

Motilal had come to my door number 13 the same evening. He had come to warn me. I dare not impress his girl anymore in future. Otherwise . . . and otherwise . . . Many otherwises gathered into one common otherwise, which was, he would not let me live in peace if I tried it again. He could bleed me to death or he could pour hot tea from my own kettle on my head, or he could invite all the monkeys to jump on my tin roof all night. And everything had the root in those harmless earrings with the red glass beads.

Manju was not bothered. She kept walking up and down the lanes of the Refugee Colony, wearing those earrings, showing them off to anybody and everybody. She even showed herself at the rickshaw stand more frequently that day.

I did not argue with Motilal because every man in his place could feel threatened although I had no such intention whatsoever. I had just given those earrings to Manju because they would suit no one other than her.

When he had exhausted all his energy and curses, I offered him a mug of tea. He accepted my gift and talked about his dead ram. He also spoke about his hopes, which were growing bigger with each word of his. It took him higher, away from the dust which lay all around him.

And the red glass bead earrings of Manju remained in my heart like her flashing smile, which was also beyond the dust in some unreachable height.

Jasmines

> And then under the starlit sky
> When the jasmines bloom
> And the heart of mine feels
> Lonely like the moon

The shadow of the night holds many secrets. Secret thoughts, secret of the silence and secret of darkness.

And those secrets can be revealed to you, if you try to stand behind the wall of the house belonging to Ramiya's widow and strain your ears in the silence. You can hear the jasmine bush which has grown near her door. You can hear her breaths which spread in the air along with the fragrance of the jasmines. You can be sure that the flowers are communicating with each other, if you are lucky enough to hear strange whispers.

Ramiya's widow knows about it. So she comes out at that time in her white widow's attire, when the moon shines white and lonely, scattering some of its secrets along with its white light. Her face reflecting all that secret in those lonely moments. She does not talk while I slowly come near her to sit by her in silence, careful not to disturb the whispering jasmines. I sit there with the night maturing around me till everything including Ramiya's widow becomes a part of the night. She sits in the same place with her own secrets while the night thrives around us.

> And yet those nights I yearn to see
> And in its moonlight I wait to be
> When the secrets are about me
> So are the moonbeams, so is she.

For a long while, the jasmines smell as nothing else but jasmines. But after a while I realize that they are getting mixed up with other smells, like that of the big drain behind the Refugee Colony. I know I have to come back inside my door number 13, for some secrets shall never be unfolded even if I wait for the whole night.

I leave her by the jasmine bush to continue the night.

Echoing Names

> And my very own names
> With my shadow they all remain
> For they echo in silence
> In my ears again and again

The morning was a restless one for me. It needed some reason to be restless. But the reason could not be any exact one.

For it could be the dusty sky
It could be my sleepless night
It could be the mosquito bite
Could be that boy on the road side.

And that boy was any boy who was picking rags. He had his little shadow following him, which was also picking up shadow rags from the scattered garbage. And my shadow reminded me that it used to follow me around every morning once upon a time, when it was of the same size as that boy's shadow. It picked up shadow rags while I picked up rags.

The whole morning and the whole afternoon my bag gave me time to fill it up. I watched its shadow getting bigger and bigger as it got filled with plastic bottles, tin cans, and other etceteras. In the evening we all, my shadow, myself, my bag's shadow, and my bag, went to the trader who sat at the entrance of the market. He paid me for those bottles and tins.

I had never starved. And I had never saved. I spent everything I got. When my stomach had enough, I bought jasmines from the woman who sat at the entrance of the temple and sold those merrygold garlands and lots of white jasmines. I spent all my remaining coins on jasmines. I bought them for me and nobody else.

I kept them near me when I slept under the cart of Mamoon Miaan.

I saw the boy again. What does he do with the money he gets? Does he buy jasmines? I plucked some jasmines from the bush which grew by the house of Ramiya's widow and offered them to the little boy. The boy had looked at me in a strange way and clumsily took the flowers. He did not know what to do with them. So he kept them in his bag along with those plastic bags and bottles.

I did not wait there anymore. The morning was around me with the usualness. I tried to blend my restlessness with its usualness.

I had to hurry to the factory gate. The tea break was at nine.

Summer Wind

> Summer wind had blown the dust
> Some of it had entered my heart
> To rush my memories some years back
> On those yellow desert tracks.

Rabbia the gypsy girl used to chase the wind on those dust-filled summer afternoons, when the desert sands yearned to become a part of the wind.

Rabbia became a part of the wind too, as she hopped

and skipped on the sand dunes with her copper-coloured feet, wearing her orange skirt on those yellow noons.

And I chased her with my turban tied around my head, which usually blew off in the wind.

Then she followed my turban and I followed her.

The wind followed everything.

I had bought her the trinkets to tie around her waist, so that whenever she chased the wind, they would tinkle with their little bells around her copper waist. Soft tinkles with her soft giggles. Soft giggles with the soft sound of the flying sand.

Our footsteps getting marked on the sand. The foot-marks getting wiped by the settling dust, replacing those marks by the beautiful striped furrow marks of the wind, shadowed by the summer sun.

"What is your name?" she had asked.

"What would you like to call me?" I had asked.

She called me Rabu. And I called myself Rabu the gypsy.

I followed the gypsy camp wherever Rabbia went.

I had learnt the art of calling the desert hawks by whistling in a particular way. The birds would perch on my shoulder, and I had to feed them with pieces of dead rats and desert snakes.

Rabbia had taught me how to track a snake by its mark on the sand. How to follow it to the hole and then, how to hold its neck when it came out of the hole irritated by the smoke shown at the mouth of the hole.

"You should be fast enough to hold its neck and chop off its head before the reptile fights back.

"Share with the hawks and the tribe."

She would say many things and I would do many things.

> And so my days
> Were coloured by her ways
> And when the colouring was done
> I walked again
> For a different name
> My shadow was followed by none.

> And wind had blown many a time
> Yet no one followed it
> Like those I had left
> On the Desert's breast
> Those copper running feet.

Here under the margossa tree, when the leaves sway in the summer wind and when dust grains rise up by the wind, I just watch it.

I never even try to chase anything, because I am no more Rabu the gypsy, following Rabbia, who wears her orange skirt and trinkets and runs with her copper feet on those yellow noons.

All Common Things

> Crows and ants are common things
> Like the dust and stones
> So they all are left unseen
> And are left alone.

The branches of the margossa tree fill up with crows during teatimes. While after teatimes crews of little ants appear to feed on the pieces and crumbs of buns and biscuits which lie scattered under the margossa tree like those little grains of dust.

Crows are too common even to get a second look. So nobody is really bothered about their presence over their heads or on the tin shed of the Favourite Tea Shop. Perhaps all those men who stand or sit around under the tree to drink tea look equally common to those birds. So they are never afraid of those men.

Hence one of those crows came near Haribai some moment when he was discussing some problem with Ramdin. And then it came nearer and closer. Perhaps it was ignored because it was only a crow. The presence of the bird was felt, however, when it had snatched a biscuit from Haribai's lap.

And everyone realized that there were too many crows around. And then what? All those men around became careful with their own pieces of snacks. I saw the other crows fighting over the piece of biscuit on the dust, blowing dust with their wings.

Haribai rebuked me when he saw me generously throwing some of the biscuits which were with me towards those birds, because Hussain and Ali had laid their bets on the winner bird already.

"How could you encourage biscuit snatching of a bird?

"And how could you encourage men gambling over it?"

I did not argue with Haribai because customers are always right.

And Haribai was so impressed by the humble tea seller that he bought one more biscuit from me. He took a full two minutes to eat it, this time showing them to those birds, challenging them to come and try snatching it from him again. He was not bothered about Ramdin and Hussain teasing him.

And those birds watched with disinterest. They never teased.

When the break was over, the birds flew away one by one, leaving the rest to the ant crew to finish. I was left alone with the dust once again. And when the last bird was ready to take off, I threw a biscuit piece towards it.

Good and Bad

Good and bad are linked with selves
Though they seem apart

> Just like day links with night
> At the hour of dusk.

I was arguing with myself about a suitable name for me before reaching Ashoknagar. It is always difficult to argue with your own self, because none of your conflicting sides can be humbled easily.

I was standing in a big field of names around me. Names ranged from Munshi and Alladin, to Kishore and Rakhalal. Some names like Narendra Nath were too sophisticated for me, although I wanted to have a name like that. Finally I chose Mukund. It suited my thin shadow.

> And my name remained with me
> When I entered the new city
> While I walked the roads and the lanes
> Trying to find a new acquaintance.

And then I saw the good and bad.

The good was the jasmine bush which had the white flowers blooming by the door of Ramiya's widow in the hour of the dusk. The good was Ramiya's widow offering me water on hearing that I was thirsty. The good was her smile which had something in common with those blooming flowers and the soft darkness around.

And the bad was my nagging reminder that I was Shamlal the thief. The bad was the hopes of mine, which tried to seek something more from her hospitality. And the bad was my evil eye of Shamlal the thief, which kept wondering about what could be hidden inside the big chest of her room.

"What is your name?" she had asked.

I was so involved with my thoughts of Shamlal the thief that I had replied, "Shamlal."

I immediately rectified myself and told, "Mukund."

She had smiled and said, "Never mind your name or who you are or what you shall call yourself. I shall arrange a place for you to stay."

Did she find out that I was never called Mukund? Maybe she came to know that I was never given any name.

I never asked. She never told.

She trusted me.

It was she who had given me a loan to start my tea trade. She took the money out from her chest right in front of my eyes. My eyes vowed never to become the eyes of Shamlal the thief again.

> And thus the good and the bad
> Were linked with the bond of trust
> As links twilight in the dark,
> With daylight by its touch.

She had arranged my stay in the Refugee Colony. She had referred me to the owner of the colony as a trusted relative.

The jasmines bloomed every night to remind me that I still had to pay the loan back to her.

The loan of trust.

All Those Dust

> And all the grains of dust in feet
> And the dust I breathe
> All those dust I step on which
> Lay countless around indeed.

I do not count all the good things which I have met on my way sometimes as Mukund, sometimes as Rahamatullah, and sometimes as Shamlal, although I recall them. I do not count the bad things either. For I have been good and bad with all my names.

However, when I sit and watch the hole of my room through which the smell of the drain enters during those damp days, I can see all those good and bad sides of each of my names.

I see Shamlal snatching a chain from the woman, who was not at all aware of it until two minutes later, in a crowded bus. I see Habib being a pretend tourist guide, explaining to the tourists some made-up story of his own. Again I see myself as Rahamatullah the rickshaw puller, returning a purse to the owner, tracking his address from a paper kept inside the purse after a full day's search.

I recalled my days when I worked as a porter in the Jagatpur Forest bungalow where I had learnt how to read and write.

> Some dust is thrown out to dust
> Those which stick to feet
> While the dust which clings to my names
> Is yet not emptied.
> Little grains sticking to heart
> With its very beats
> And so perhaps I walk on earth
> Still with dust on feet.

So while I keep my eye on the hole of my room, I see those grains of dust floating on the air, entering me through my nostrils. I allow them to be a part of my breaths. And they allow me to be a part of themselves.

Forest Days

> Mystery hid in the murmuring wind
> Mystery in her looks
> Mystery in the forest green
> Mystery in an unread book
> And those mysteries one by one
> Gathered with knots of some kind
> Like a twine that binds the thoughts
> In my secret mind.

How old was I then? I was not a man. I was not a boy either. I was still a self-named person. And others called me what I wanted them to call me.

I came to live in the Jagatpur Forest bungalow as a porter. When I had got bored with the wine shop on the highway, where I worked and lived, I decided to change my everythings. My everythings included my name, identity, and also my work. Malu, the truck driver, had helped me to come to the forest bungalow.

Malu had known me since the past year because the wine shop was on his way to the forest. He usually parked his truck there to relax his muscles and senses. He carried timber from the forest to the paper mill on the Madhopura district. He usually boasted of being a very close friend to the forest officer posted there.

He had gladly given me a free lift to the forest, telling the guards that I was a distant cousin. I got the job as a porter in the guest house. During the evenings, I worked as a servant in the bungalow of the forest officer.

"Do you want to read?" his daughter had asked me when she saw me turning through the pages of her magazine.

I do not remember whether I had nodded or not because I was indifferent to anything which people with names sticking to them aspire to. And what exactly should I do with myself after learning to read? I kept quiet because I did not know whether I really needed to read. I did not require to write even a letter to anybody like Kusumlal, who wrote every month to his wife.

She thought that I was interested to read.

I was slow to learn. She was hopeful and persistent.

Slowly I began to read the words and then the sentences.

And one day I got tired of everything and I turned once again to the roads. The road took me from the narrow forest tracks to the dusty lanes and then to the wider world made of more dust. The green shade of the trees opened into the wider world of sunshine.

I had carried nothing with me, except for a thick book from her shelf, of the house as a memory. I would never be able to read those big words, but I would at least be able to touch them over and over again.

It would remind me of her because often I had seen her touching those words while reading them.

It was her favourite book.

Back with the Dust Grains

> A little of shine, and a little of rain
> A little of me, and my all those names
> Like dust fields, and little dust grains
> While my shadow is yet the same.

What mattered more to me now were all those loads of names. All those names belonging to me either in Ashoknagar or Jhumripur or under the roof of a roadside food shop. Like those little grains of dust which were already there within me because I had breathed them in me.

Dust grains which stuck to my feet could be washed easily in the corporation tap or with the water of a temple well or with the water from Kashiram's borewell. While all those dust grains which entered my blood stream remained within me.

So when Ramdin calls his son as Shamlal, I feel that he is calling me.

So when old Hukumat Begam mentions her dead

brother, I feel that she is mentioning me, because her brother was also named Habib.

> Dust grains are too common
> And are everywhere
> They fly and travel all along
> In land and in the air.
> Grains of dust are so common
> They fly with the summer wind
> When they fall in the eyes
> Tears of dust they bring.

And once more I long to go searching for some dust grains which I have lost on my way.

The dust grains which remained on the wheels of Rahamatullah's rickshaw.

The dust grains which marked my footsteps on the yellow noons of a desert on which those copper-coloured feet of Rabbia used to run.

The dust grains which remained back in Jhumripur and now in Ashoknagar under the margossa tree where I sold my tea to Surkhiram and Hussain and Ramdin and Dayal. And all those dust grains which flew around with the quarreling crows' wing-flappings, during the nine o'clock tea breaks.

And once more
I was on the road
Carrying my emptiness
With a little of sun and
A little of shade
To seek a new place.

I had carried nothing with me, except the night jasmines which I had plucked from the bush which grew by the door of Ramiya's widow. I had never turned back to see because I knew that she was listening to the dark night and the blooming jasmines.

Some things are allowed to get lost.

The Broken Mirror

"The Broken Mirror" was written when I was fourteen years old. I loved watching through mirrors since I was a little boy. I did not know anything about the laws of reflection then. I believed that there was a parallel world behind any mirror which was as real as the world where I stood. I often wondered what mirrors thought of this world. Thus was born "The Broken Mirror."

One

The broken mirror is the only object in the room with which the lonely room can interact.

All the other objects, like the rocking chair, the marble table, the ancient faces of the forgotten people with their stilled eyes on the portraits hanging on the walls all around the room with gathering dust grains, the high carved ceiling with a few cobwebs in the corner, and the rusting iron on the window grills, are the mute observers of the stilled time inside the room and moving time outside the room.

The broken mirror is the only face which shows the room how it slowly got that withered look. Slowly through the days. Slowly through the years.

✻   ✻   ✻

The room all around the mirror, part by part, could classify its sides as the northern side with the two large wall murals of the winged fairies, which always face each other and never bother to look at the mirror, perhaps because they see the image of each other in each other's faces, the eastern side with the large window with rust on the grills which shows the sun peeping behind the old jackfruit tree, where a couple of crows sit in the afternoons to discuss "God knows what," the western side with the large oak door which opens once in the festival of the summer solstice and then closes for the rest of the year, and the southern side, the image of which is impossible for the room to see because the mirror hangs from the southern wall.

The broken mirror stays in that central position on the southern wall, with a kind of satisfied stability, ever since this room was built, except for those times when the room gets cleaned or whitewashed, every five years, when the owners of this house fancy.

And the rest of the year the forgotten mirror in the forgotten room of this ancestral house remains in a close state of a deep conspiracy with the whole room, with the four boundaries of the walls, the carved ceiling, and also the checked floor, with alternate arrangement of marble and granite slabs, always mocking the ceiling with a sense of probable pride for its valued stones, which the ceiling can never even get to touch.

A state of a deep conspiracy and a secret mocking for everything which has submitted to the changing of time, trying to keep up with the speed of the outside world.

Nothing could touch the spirit of this confined room and the spirit of the broken mirror. Not even the old wall clock which could be heard from this room, as the house-keeper never forgets to turn on its keys, even on the raining nights before turning the light of the hall off.

The broken mirror hears the sound of the clock bell with a mocking deep concern. It knows very well that nothing else will happen that night, except for the passing-away moments.

Everything remains the same.

And the clock strikes nine.

Two

The sun was lighting the outside world with a flood of the July light. There were different kinds of sounds coming from the old jackfruit tree and the outside earth.

The sound of a constant wind rippling past the leaves, reorienting its direction as the air particles got tossed by each leaf, the sounds of the group of sparrows which started to quarrel just for the sake of quarrelling, the softer sound of the ticks of the clock from somewhere in some room which could only be heard if you cared to hear it, and the fainter sound of the breaths of the earth, which only the broken mirror can hear and the old jackfruit tree can hear because its roots can feel the breathing of the earth, somewhere deep below their limits to reach.

The breaths of joy, the breaths of pain, and the breaths of indifference, which the broken mirror can understand as the jackfruit tree can detect the ripples of the earth's every breath to get reflected by the broken face of the mirror.

The sounds of a distant market with a constant collective echo reaching the peripheries of the room and stealing its way inside if you carefully listened, the sound of a buzzing fly which happened to enter through the window and knocked against the mirror, making the mistake over and over again, thinking that the reflection of the window was its way to the outside world, the sound of the stilled breath of the very room wanting to exhale out a still breath which got stuck in its own boundaries, and the very sound of the silent dust grains on the floor which try to exchange their positions because they do not like to be in the same place for long, all get reflected by the broken mirror.

And the broken mirror echoes back those sounds for the whole room to echo back.

Once, twice, and thrice.

Till all those sounds become one collective sound. The very sound of loneliness.

Three

Nothing in the enclosed room could show any reason why the room could feel that the broken mirror was reflecting the image of a rainy evening when a frightened sparrow had entered the room, perhaps lost, or perhaps to find a shelter there.

There was the July sunshine outside, and there was the dry spell of a prolonged dry rainless month since the past two months. Then why should the event of the rainy evening be replayed behind the broken mirror's face?

The room watched the sparrow dripping with water, a little miserable creature of bones and feathers, trying to limp and then trying to fly.

The room watched everything happening behind the broken mirror's face.

The bird, darting straight across the room and being deceived by the image of the window behind the mirror, heading straight towards it, and then knocking its beak on the surface of the mirror, startled at first but then regaining the confidence and going back towards it to give another try and getting knocked by its own darting reflection, and then trying once again to be knocked back.

There was nothing the room could do to help the bird. There was nothing the mirror could do either.

The sparrow had been too attached to its own reflection. Perhaps was threatened by it. Perhaps had fallen in love with it. The secret behind its coming back could never be known to anybody. And there was nothing the room could do. The earth had begun to turn dark for the night to grow and spread.

There was the attraction of the image.
There was the spreading darkness growing around the room.
There was the fear of losing sight of its image.
There was the desperate flying, knocking and trying again.
And then there was tiredness.
There was fear.

Then there was night.
And then there was hunger.
A little squeak and trying to fly.
Then all was silent.

The mirror reflected that prolonged silence of that evening.
While a bright July day waited to be reflected.

Four

Happy times.

Summer days bring in happy times inside the whole room, on the walls, the rocking chair, the marble table, and the broken mirror's oxidised copper frame.

The floor, with its alternate square slabs of marble and granite, waits with warm friendliness for those footsteps to enter the room.

The ceiling, with those cobwebs, waits to be cleared of all those insects which got entrapped in those meshes of complicated latticework.

The two mural fairies too must wait, while they face each other and see the eagerness reflect in each other's eyes.

The broken mirror gets a polish.

The housekeeper's wife scrubs its oxidised copper frame vigorously yet very carefully. She is always careful with the diagonal broken line, which divides any reflection into two parts.

The parts show more distinctly when the distance increases.

The walls of the room are usually seen in two parts through the mirror. But they never complain.

✻   ✻   ✻

When you get used to seeing yourself through something, and when you see it like that over and over again, and when you know that complaining will not change anything, you take things for granted. Even distortion is overlooked when you get used to it. The mirror too has got used to the diagonal broken line which had made its surface bisect anybody's face if he stood in front of it right in the middle. The faces too must have got used to seeing their reflections in that bisecting way.

So no one complains.

In fact, one of the bigger boys, who gets bigger and taller every year when he visits this ancestral home before the festival of summer solstice, picks up each of the younger cousins to show them their faces through the broken mirror.

Some children are amused. Some are too frightened because the bigger brother tells them that is how their faces will become if they do not obey him.

And then everything becomes a part of the festival of the summer solstice as relatives and more relatives come, one by one, to fill the house and this room with laughter and happiness.

The broken mirror listens to them, reflecting those happy sounds.

The walls of the room echo them back for the rest of the year, to repeat through the years. Years of preserved memories.

And all those memories get enclosed somewhere inside the depths of the walls, where there are secret cracks, which grow with the years.

And all those memories are kept within the spaces between the old rocking chair where the oldest member of this family sits with his grandchildren flocking around and the marble table where he keeps his silver-rimmed spectacles and his case of cigarettes.

The mirror knows that after some years, he will be replaced by someone else.

And then by someone else.

As the cracks of the wall will not remain secrets anymore, like an aging woman's growing furrows of wrinkles, there will be more faces to add and replace the older ones.

Perhaps some faces will turn into portraits and hang on the walls of some room, just as a reminder that they had once filled this house with their laughter.

And happy times return with summer. The broken mirror is included.

Five

Everyone waits for the summer solstice with great eagerness, including the broken mirror. It hears the housekeeper's wife entering the room opening the big oak door with the heavy bunch of keys.

It waits for her bangles to tinkle as she keeps her heavy bunch of keys on the marble table. And then her bangles tinkle more and more while she starts polishing the woodwork of the chair and on the legs of the marble table with the polish she bring with her. She clears the cobwebs with her long broom and dusts every corner where those little dust grains get too stubborn to be removed. She stares at those wall portraits for some time, wondering about who those faces could belong to, and then wipes them clean to get a clearer view of them.

The mirror has seen her since the past two years. Before her, there was a different woman. And before that different woman, there was someone else. The mirror knows that one day she will be replaced by a new face. It wonders where those old faces go.

But now the mirror is not concerned about that.

It knows that it will get a good polish. The housekeeper's wife usually keeps it waiting. Polishing it is her last task. She needs to dust the windows and clear the rust settled on the grill first.

Only then can she turn towards the mirror.

It is a big moment for the broken mirror. It is unhooked from the big nail and placed on the floor very carefully. She hugs the mirror and the mirror can feel the beat of her heart so close to it.

Moments are counted with those heartbeats. Those precious moments holding in the reflection of the broken mirror while it wishes to hold them for ever in its own heart if it had one.

The housekeeper's wife starts polishing the oxidised copper frame by carefully scraping the green oxidised copper. Then she rubs the frame with some waxlike substance, which has a very strong smell. The mirror feels her gentle hands and hears her bangles while she works on the frame before polishing the glass.

The broken mirror reflects her face back to her while she tries to wipe a pearl-like sweat drop from her forehead.

Six

There are times when each and every thing is new. So there was a time when this house was new too. So was the mirror, which was not broken when it was first brought to this house by the then master of this house. So was the new smell of this room, which was so distinct to the mirror when it was first hung. So was the young jackfruit tree, which could then barely reach the top of the roof.

There was so much sunshine around the house and so much to wait for. The room would wait for the daily cleaning. The floor would wait for getting a polish so that the marble would show whiter and the granite slabs would show darker against the marble. The master of this house would see a scratch on the floor and order someone to polish it again.

The mirror would also get a cleaning. The frame would show the reddish shine of copper instead of the dull oxidised green patches. And the master of this house would personally stand in front of it and look through it, perhaps towards the future which he knew that the mirror would one day show.

The broken mirror could show him the future if it knew about it.

And the broken mirror could show him all those faces, whoever they belonged to, if at all it could know them as it does now.

The broken mirror shows the walls the slow cracks on them. It also shows the walls how they looked when this house was new. Everything can be seen through the broken mirror if you have the memory and the imagination to see it.

Memories are all kept with care behind its vast memory-scape.

Seven

There could be many things to wait for.

Waiting for the next moment or waiting for the sum of all those moments, which could be added together as future moments. Then waiting for a forgotten moment to flash out in the present moment, like some forgotten faces whose voices could echo in the room by those walls, which the mirror could not recall.

And then showing the walls a face whose voice still waits to be recalled by the walls to echo back and bring out the memory of the person in completeness when he actually was a part of the moment.

There are waiting moments like the coming of a new leaf when all the leaves of the jackfruit tree have been shed as a part of the annual ritual of nature. The jackfruit tree has told the mirror that every deciduous tree has to go through this annual ritual of shedding old leaves. The jackfruit tree tells the mirror many things about the outside world, which the mirror could never see. For instance, there is the field across which there is the railway track. And the trains run on those railway tracks. The broken mirror has heard those trains come and go. They come and go twice a day. It does not matter which is the direction of coming or going to the broken mirror.

But the old jackfruit tree has reassured it that when the sound travels from north to south, it is the sound of the train coming. And if the sound travels from south to north, then be sure that it is the sound of a train going.

How does the train look?

The broken mirror has often wondered. The jackfruit tree has wondered too, with its natural blindness. There is no way by which it could show the mirror what the train looks like. Its powerful whistle proves that the train is no small object. It is sure that the train is something long. Long like that snake, which curves its way from the house towards the field as it coils around the bark of the tree as its evening ritual. The jackfruit tree cannot guess where it goes.

The train could be heard from one point of the horizon to another point, and so the jackfruit tree can well understand that the train is much bigger than the snake.

The broken mirror tries to picture the train as well as the snake.

The jackfruit tree talks about the field where the mound lies, burying under it all the secrets of the earth. The jackfruit tree is sure that the earth stores all its secrets under that mound. There is no reason as to why the mound should be there when the rest of the field around is so flat.

The tree has heard the cowherds playing on the mound during those idle winter afternoons when the wind begins to blow from the south, bringing with it the smells from the distant market, which cannot be seen from the house.

The cowherds play "king and subjects" on the mound. They choose a king for the day, and the rest of them become subjects. The king settles fake disputes, while the subjects bring in complaints like stolen cows and not paying the right amount for a cow which can milk twice as much as any cow found on the earth.

The king has the right to punish the way he wants to.

Like walking on the hands by keeping the feet up and balancing for two minutes, or running across the field and coming back before he counts ten, or carrying the king on his back and pretending to be a horse.

The king for the day may turn into offender for the next day, as he may have to face a similar punishment by the next day's king.

The mirror hears the stories from the outside world from the jackfruit tree and stores them behind its infinite space.

There are more stories to wait for. All those stories seen only through imaginations if you happened to stand in front of the broken mirror.

Eight

Many things can happen in a day. And one of those things can change your appearance forever.

The jackfruit tree, for instance, began to look so different when most of its branches on the lower part were chopped in the rainy month of August. And all the day there was panic amongst those little sparrows as they saw the branches being chopped off. The jackfruit tree had begun to look so different.

Yet slowly everyone got used to looking at the jackfruit tree with the chopped-off branches, after some days. Even the little sparrows, which had made such a loud protest, had got used to it.

It took the broken mirror just a moment's time to get that crack.

And that moment came one day. There were many events around this room that day. Many happy events.

A ceremony was taking place. People were coming in and going out of this room. There were children, too, running in and running out.

The mirror showed everyone what they wanted to see. Those who wanted to see their faces could see them through it, as they wanted their faces to be. Those who wanted to see themselves beautiful saw themselves as beautiful through the mirror. Those who wanted to see themselves younger used the mirror to apply some touches of dye to their hair borders, when no one was watching, till they were satisfied.

The mirror never disappointed anyone.

There were many faces coming and going to and from the mirror. And all those faces got reflected back as best the mirror could show.

But moments can create any event. And events are plenty to happen.

One of the boys had darted into the room that day, chased by another boy. The mirror showed their coming reflections to them. They were not bothered about their shadows. They were a part of some chasing game, as boys of their ages are supposed to play.

The mirror saw them dodging each other around the marble table and gaining speed.

And then it happened. As anything needs just a moment to happen, it needed just a moment.

One of the boys knocked against the mirror, bringing it down as it fell on the ground, along with the startled boy.

After that nothing was the same.

The mirror was hung up, but there were fewer faces to see themselves through it, other than some idle stray looks.

Children, however, got interested with it more than ever. The bigger boys scared the smaller ones by showing their images through the broken mirror, threatening them about how their faces would turn if the mirror got really angry.

The broken mirror hangs on the wall staring at the moments.

Happy moments and lonely moments, wondering how their images would look.

Nine

There was a storm last evening. And some of the drops of the wild rain had entered into the room through the window.

Summer storms are like fresh breaths of nature, because they bring in so much momentum to the suffocation of the still air around.

Just before it began raining, there was a dust storm. The jackfruit tree had swayed with the wind, dancing with the tune of nature. It had let off some old leaves which had flown farther and farther away, competing with the flying dust, ready to go anywhere. Even the earth seemed ready to fly, as the wind around the mound picked up some loose dust grains, creating a huge bowl of whirling brown impatient dust.

The sound of the jackfruit tree branches, the sound of the distant dust storm, approaching towards the house, the sound of the windowpane banging in some room, and the sound of the confused birds on the tree had set up a sound of celebration of its own kind. Nature in the form of wind was enjoying its power, turning the earth into a ground of celebration.

The broken mirror, from its stilled position, heard the sound of celebration with silence and wonder. How should the earth look like when it celebrated its own power?

And along with the broken mirror, the room wondered too. It was so bounded by its own enclosed walls, limiting it into a finite size. The only eye of the room was the window, which brought in shadows of the swaying branches of the jackfruit tree, ready to get reflected by the broken mirror.

Some stray dust grains entered through the window. Those dust grains settled down anywhere they found a place to settle. They could never be settled in one place for a long time. At the slightest provocation of a light breeze, they would exchange places.

How much the broken mirror wished that it could be like those free dust particles and go anywhere with the wild wind. How much it wished to see the beyonds of the jackfruit leaves which swayed just outside the window. Perhaps it could settle down on the mound, which the jackfruit tree talks about and where the earth hides all its secrets. Perhaps it could race across the field and try to fly with the speed of the train, showing the train how it looked. And perhaps it could one day find its way back into the enclosed walls of this room and show it all those reflections it had collected while it ran free with the wind.

The dust grains were slowly settling down on its surface, layer by layer, and reflecting themselves, making the reflections of the walls more and more dusty.

And then the raindrops had made their way as the wind entered the room through the window.

The dry summer day bathed outside the room with carefree celebration.

Ten

Darkness had come in many times to spread all around the room, entering through the open window when the sun glides west. It comes in every day as a ritual. It never hesitates to fill the corners of the floor and then spread throughout the other spaces of the room, even when there is a faint glow of the light showing in the outside sky.

Darkness enters into the room through the little space below the closed door. And then slowly covers the rest of the wall, climbing higher and higher to touch the ceiling. It seems as if all the darkness settles down inside the room before radiating out on the open world outside the open window. Yet there remains some light inside the shadows of darkness when anyone looks through the broken mirror. And the broken mirror stays awake all through the darkness to tell its many stories to anyone who cares to look at them through it.

Stories grow with darkness. And the walls of the room echo back those stories as they hear or see them. Stories travel outside the window to the branches of the jackfruit tree. And stories are passed on to the outside earth, perhaps to reach the dream of some lonely traveller who happens to rest by the mound under the starlit sky. And those stories are collected by the earth, which hides some of those stories under its mound on the open field where the cowherds play "king and subjects" on the winter afternoons.

The earth hides those stories along with its many secrets below the mound.

Some stories escape everything. They escape the lonely traveller's dream, they escape the mound on the field where the earth hides its secrets and travel further, with some free grain of dust, to reach the other side of the earth, where the sun shows daylight.

Perhaps they would return one day back to the room, with a gush of wind of a summer storm, and settle down on the very surface of the broken mirror. And all those "perhaps stories" collect together with the darkness and together with the evolving "other stories" to spread wherever they can.

Eleven

In some room, across the wall, the sound of the clock striking midnight could be heard. And in some room across the many walls, a wall lizard ticked six times to show that it was wide awake. Not many rooms beyond, footsteps could be heard. Footsteps coming from memories to visit the present moments. And footsteps going further and further across with the ticks of the clock, going across the limits of present moment.

Each moment is a captive of its own limits. Its limits of bounding time, the limits of its own capturing events.

The event of a summer solstice is so bounded with the interval of happiness. It begins with a happy moment and yet ends with a specific moment of loneliness. After the summer solstice, the room is bounded back to the lonely moments, with its hollow lonely echoing space.

Everything gets bounded by something or other. Even the field on which the mound lies, where the earth hides all its secrets, is bounded by its size. Even the heaven around the earth is the captive of some universal law which holds the stars in the space.

This room where the broken mirror lies is a captive of its own walls. And the broken mirror too lies a prisoner of its own space on the wall, limiting its images to the spaces of this room.

Do dreams, too, have boundaries? The broken mirror tries to dream the limitless. And all those limitless spaces show the absoluteness of nothing. What else to dream other than the finiteness of the validity of your own imaginations?

So the broken mirror tries to dream beyond the limits of the room with wonder-filled imaginations leading to larger doubts about the validity of those imagined dreams. And so its broken face reflects those dreams with every distortion, like its own limited ability to show a perfect image. So when it dreams of a distant star in a moonless sky, it gets a probable view of it, with the limits of a few possibilities which it can imagine. So when it dreams of the clock beating away the moments, it can just hear its beats, as its dream cannot reach the image of the clock.

The night continues to carry those beating moments away and away. The broken mirror chases them with its incomplete, broken dreams.

The Corner Shop

In Bangalore, India, where I spent several years of my life, there happened to be a shop at the corner of two streets. I called it the Corner Shop. I saw some regular visitors there who seemed to spend much of their day in that shop. I could never know what they talked about, but I could imagine some interactions. I happened to write this piece to thank those familiar strangers.

There is a corner shop on the road.

The road stretches from the bus stop at the west end till the women's college at the east end. Not exactly the east end, as we call it, because the road has never been what you call in geometry a straight line. The east end is somewhat the northeast end, considering the geographical directions. We call it the east end corner, and are quite comfortable that way.

And because we call it the east end corner, the shop is named the East End Shop.

We come to the East End Shop during the day to spend the day there. This is because it is the only place on the road that gives a proper view of the women's college. The high walls that hold the college in its secured boundary never give any opportunity to peep inside. And there is no question of climbing the walls and having a look inside, because if you did that, what would people think about you?

No one would believe you if you told them that you had your harmless intentions of satisfying your quest about the student who wore a red dress and carried a purple bag.

"Which year does she belong to?

"What happened after she entered the college?

"Who are her friends?

"And is she the most talkative girl in her batch?"

Questions cannot be answered without peeping. And how can you find your peace when you don't know anything about her?

So we come to this corner shop from where we can get a part of the view of the mysterious campus of the women's college. The gate of the college faces the corner shop. The East End Shop.

However, if you positioned yourself well, you could get a better view.

To position yourself well, you need to come earlier than the others. As early as seven A.M., when Bhoopati opens the shop and prays to the pictures of the gods to bless his shop. Otherwise you could lose your stand on the highest staircase of the shop, just at its entrance.

It would be occupied otherwise by Viru.

Viru is Bhoopati's nephew. Once he occupies the place, it would be very difficult for any of us to know what is going on inside, and what Viru would be seeing. Viru would not leave his stand. He would however give such secret smiles that they would make us wonder about the cause. He would never tell us why he smiled when the college bell rang.

There was no point asking him about it, because he would be so lost in that smile of his and the "reason for that smile of his" that our question would remain unanswered.

Viru would pretend that he had not heard us.

What could you do during this background of suspense, when the suspense is caused by Viru's smile?

Complain to Bhoopati?

That would not work. It is Bhoopati who has spoiled Viru. Because, when Viru's father died, leaving Viru in the cradle without his mother, who had died a year before, it was Bhoopati who had promised the dying man that he would take every care of the child. Viru had started getting spoiled through the stages as he grew up.

Again, it is here in Bhoopati's shop that we discuss everything.

Everything includes everything.

High-heel sandals, purple hair clips, prime minister. Purple hair clips again and the latest hit movie, our unemployed status, purple hair clips again, cigarettes, and purple hair clips once more.

We offer our suggestions about the recent Women's Bill.

Just when we think that we could get a bit intellectual by giving our views about the Political Degradation of our country, because one of us had suggested that the best way to escape unemployment is by joining Politics, first as an ordinary political worker and then a leader — simple as that, we would hear the college bell.

We would become attentive once more.

We would become attentive again because we would like to know what happens when the bell rings in a women's college.

Then we would like to know what can happen in a women's college five minutes after the bell rings.

And then what may happen fifteen minutes after that.

"Can you see the girl in the pink dress?" Abdul asks Ravi, who is the tallest among us. Nobody asks Viru anything anymore because we know that he would not tell anything. He would pretend not to hear any question, because he would be concentrating very hard from his stand. So we ask Ravi.

"Which colour dress did you ask for?" Ravi wants to know again. "Yes, I can see a green dress very clearly," he answers, standing on his toes now, trying to grow taller.

"Not green, silly.

"It is a pink dress. Rose pink." Abdul had to be precise because Ravi could forget again.

"I can see one, two, three, four — four pink-dressed girls from here," Ravi answers.

"Short hair, brown eyes, yellow sandals, and rose pink dress." Abdul gives the details.

"Blue dress, purple hair clip, plaited hair, and diamond nose stud." I give my details.

"Red-dressed, fair-faced, black eyes, matching hair clip." Ramu gives his details.

Murari gives his, and then Babu gives his details.

An old customer walks in the shop that time. Mr. Jeevan.

Everyone here knows him. He was in the police service before. Now he is retired. But he has kept his "Hitler moustache" intact even after his retirement. We respect him.

So we try to discuss how the police department is not as efficient as it used to be ten years back.

Mr. Jeevan does not look impressed. He does not comment.

Mr. Jeevan does not frown and he does not smile either.

He just looks at us clustered on the staircase of the East End Shop with our faces turned towards the college though our eyes are all turned towards him. Mr. Jeevan especially looks at Ravi, who is still standing on his toes.

And then Mr. Jeevan walks out of the shop.

Ravi continues to stand on his toes.

Mr. Jeevan walks across the road and Ravi regains his posture. He finally stands on his feet.

"Now what will happen?" Ravi is worried. "Suppose he tells my father?"

"He did not understand why you were standing on your toes," Abdul tells Ravi. "Don't worry."

"He thought that you had a sprain or something like that," I assure Ravi.

"If you limp for two days the old man will be convinced," Murali suggests.

"He will come to play chess with my father this evening. What if he complains about me?" Ravi still worries.

Bhoopati the shop owner suggests he pretend to fall sick so that there is a general sympathy at home.

"And it is good to fall sick once in a while and let people fuss over you. The very advantage of falling sick is that nobody will nag you for being unemployed at home."

"You can get caught if you fake having fever because the mercury inside the thermometer may not rise even if you wished it to," Babu had cautioned.

"So what should I fake having?" Ravi was open to all kinds of suggestions.

"Cholera."

"Yellow fever."

"Perhaps bronchitis."

"Tuberculosis." Viru was more convincing because he told Ravi that he knew how to have it. "All you have to do is cough and cough and cough."

"And see the advantage of having tuberculosis. Mr. Jeevan

Man at the Bus Stop

A man in a bus stop at the city of Bangalore made me grow my story around him. I will never know who he is, and yet I happened to feel so close to him as I saw his impatience. All the probabilities gathered around his impatience as I wrote my story.

It was not clear to me whether the man who had been standing at the bus stop by my side was in his late thirties or in his early forties. It concerned me. At least I had been concerned about him, while I did my idle waiting for my bus.

Did I have any reason to be concerned? I am not sure whether to give a justified yes or a no. But somehow I got concerned regarding him, although there were others too waiting there with me and him at the same bus stop. Perhaps his worried face, perhaps his careless kick on the stone, or perhaps his getting impatient and glancing at the watch were possible reasons.

Yet he was too ordinary. Too ordinary to stand out in the crowd. Too ordinarily dressed and too ordinarily shaped with ordinary features. And indeed a very ordinary frown on that very ordinary face showed that he had some big worry behind his ordinary frown, however ordinary that big worry was.

And his frown became my responsibility to think about. What could be his worry?

Wife? Children? Boss? Mother-in-law? Or could his own self be the cause for that worry?

What could be that self-worrying cause? Constipation? Headache? Anything else? A man like him can have a wide choice of worries.

I tried to compare his worries with our colleague Mr. Saxena's worries. Bowel problem. Saxena has taken for granted that all the problems of man begin from it. Loss of peace, concern about the next morning leading to a wakeful night followed by a row of etceteras.

I compared his worries with those of Mr. Lee. Mr. Lee, though Chinese in origin, was very much Indian at heart, his ancestors having settled down in this country as early as World War I. Mr. Lee worried about his wife's family of six sisters, who were all staying with him, waiting to get married with some suitable grooms. And those suitable grooms needed to be Chinese in blood. How should Mr. Lee find suitable blood here in this remote Rampur?

I had suggested a total migration back to Hong Kong. There would be plenty of grooms anywhere to look and choose from.

"Matrimonial advertisement," Mitra had suggested.

"Polygamy," Gupta had suggested. Mr. Lee had said that he had no objection to that, but he was doubtful whether his wife would let him go for it.

✳   ✳   ✳

I saw the man at the bus stop once again.

Did he have similar sisters-in-law, each one more suitable than the other? I was tempted once or twice to ask him and try to be friendly. Obviously he shouldn't mind that. However, I did not even try it. I hesitated. Because I wondered whether it was a "sister-in-law" problem or a "brother-in-law" problem.

"Brother-in-law" problem like the one they had shown in a movie of the sixties in which the hero was repeatedly being cheated by his brother-in-law. But he could not do anything about it because he loved his wife, and his wife loved her brother, thus forming a vicious circle.

And my imagination about the man who stood by my side at the bus stop started to run wild. The ten o'clock summer sky was already causing a lot of sweat, and with it a greater impatience. Impatience flowing down the man's forehead as sweat. "Big forehead," I observed, "What a big frown on that big forehead!"

I looked at the man once again. The man was looking at his watch now and then. He was also tapping his left knuckles with his right-hand fingers, obviously showing his impatience. The bus was nowhere around to be spotted.

Bus timings can never be guessed here in Rampur. When you are in a hurry, you may find the bus trying to teach you how to be patient. Buses teach you many more things other than patience in Rampur. They can teach you how to squeeze yourself along with others and balance your body at the same time along with the rhythm of the go, because of the potholes on the road, especially when the going gets through the Nehru Market. They teach you to stand in harmony as you knock your head and rub your shoulders with others. Coexistence and brotherhood are taught through the journey on one of these buses. And time moves with the moving bus.

Nothing is stable, however slow it may seem. Certainly time is not.

The man checked his watch once again. The summer sun reflected on the dial of the watch. A rather large dial, I observed. A jumbo dial around his slender wrist. A perfect time to start a conversation.

Perhaps with a, "Er — what is the time?" I however could not start my word because he suddenly became conscious of my peeping eyes and moved away.

Some people do not like to talk to strangers, however friendly the stranger's intentions may be.

He reminded me of my boss. Once I needed a leave during the annual inspection period. The reason was my father-in-law's annual visit. Something inside had prevented me from telling my boss the real reason for my leave application. So I had written that my grandfather had passed away as the reason for my leave application.

I was called by my boss in his office. Naturally it was my first chance to get friendly with him. I had entered with my most friendly intentions. Here I stood, and there sat he. Between us, there was only a table. My leave application on that table. And since my leave application had the reason of my grandfather's passing away, I had made a sad face. Wasn't I supposed to look sad? I have never met any grandfather because I was not even born when either had passed away.

But I was sure that my boss, whom we called "Shark Face" behind his back, would sympathise with me, seeing my sad face. Maybe he would offer his narrow shoulders to give me support if I did not hold myself at this terrible time of loss. "Shark Face will not remain a Shark Face anymore. Perhaps a more friendly Dolphin Face from now." My thoughts got interrupted.

"Which grandfather of yours has died? Paternal or maternal?"

There were two options to choose from. Time was running fast. I had no living grandfather to make my task simple. I mumbled out a "Paternal grandfather."

"I was very attached to him, sir," I continued.

I tried to make a very sad face, as sad as possible. As sad as it should be.

Shark Face did not look impressed. "I thought that your last year's leave note mentioned about a death of your grandfather." He was not sympathetic.

"Remarkable memory," I thought. But I was already in it. So I had no other options left but to convince him that it was my grandfather's brother and this brother was one amongst nine other brothers my grandfather had. Etcetera.

Etceteras got piled up to form our family tree, because that would make my boss believe my aggrieved situation.

However when my boss began to look at his watch again and again, I knew that I had to leave his room. Before leaving I had observed his watch. "Too large a dial for his wrist."

I however kept my options open about eight living brothers my grandfather still had, which would enable me to take eight leaves if they died. My boss had never given me any opportunity to get friendly after that.

Returning my thoughts back to that man waiting with his worries and impatience at the bus stop, I found him still tapping his left knuckles with his right-hand fingers, but this time the beat was faster. Which bus should he take? Was it the same bus for which I was waiting? I hoped that he joined me through my bus journey. I might get the answer as to why he looked worried.

The man started pacing up and down. I started pacing up and down with him also, to show my solidarity with him. However, since it made him irritated because he gave me a direct frown, I had to stop pacing. He chose not to be friendly after all. And my curiosity remained unsolved because my bus had arrived before his bus. I had no other option but to get on it.

As I looked out of the window I saw him standing there. And no one was left at the bus stop to watch over him.

He was anybody once again. Just a man at the bus stop. A worried man at the bus stop. With any sort of worry for me to guess about. Did I feel sorry for him? Did I feel sorry for not being able to find out about his worry? I cannot be sure. It could be because I did feel sorry.

However, everything in this world need not be known to you. That is why you are able to guess. The good thing about guessing is that you can guess anything. And anything can be everything.

Sometimes I wonder.

Sometimes I wonder about him. Are his worries the usual worries which I face? Wife, boss, children, leave application, loans, retirement, and mother-in-law? Could I have offered him any real help if I came to know of it, other than tell him not to worry? I wonder.

I wonder about the man at the bus stop.

The worried man who stood with me at the bus stop.

A somebody I would never know about.

The Calendar

I love calendars. I collect them. Mother taught me how to read numbers from a date calendar. This piece is a fond tribute to all my calendars. The calendar in this story happens to be in an office described by my cousin in India, where most of the workers were more interested in getting their paychecks at the end of the month than in working.

A calendar.

A date calendar.

A date calendar on the wall behind Mr. Basu's chair.

We come and we work. We come, work, and we go. The calendar keeps a watch at each and every one of us from the wall behind Mr. Basu's chair like the guardian angel.

Sometimes it reminds us that it is the month of March. And when we start getting used to the month of March, and being in March like the chair and the month of March, the table and the month of March, the high office ceiling and the month of March, the typewriter and the month of March, the piled-up files and the month of March, Mr. Basu's big head in front of the month of March, and peon Ravi's coming in and going out in the month of March, we suddenly find that the month of March is over and Mr. Basu has changed the page to the month of April.

It takes time. It takes time to get used to the new page of the calendar.

This is because we never looked forward to the new month. In fact we never look forward to anything that could remind us that the files of the previous month are still sitting on our tables.

And it would mean that our boss Mr. Ramapani could call one of us any time and ask for an explanation, behind the partition, where he sits.

Mr. Ramapani never smiles. Mr. Basu is sure of the fact that he would not smile even if he is tickled. Mr. Ramapani, however, opens his mouth once, when someone wishes him a "good morning."

And Mr. Ramapani sits behind the partition and opens his mouth to question us.

The calendar with its fresh set of dates reminds us of these things, which include our pending files and Mr. Ramapani's questions. Mr. Basu never will turn the page after ten days, giving us time to settle for the next month. He is too punctual to turn the pages.

So we wait every time the calendar changes the page. We wait because Mr. Wasim Khan is the first person whom Mr. Ramapani calls behind the partition. After that we get our turns to see Mr. Ramapani, whose eyebrows automatically get raised when he sits behind his table.

He questions at first and then comments about the ineffi-ciency of the present-day working class and his disappointment, because it is very difficult for him to believe that we are the citizens of the same country where Gandhi lived and breathed.

Mr. Wasim Khan, being the first person to be called inside, has the opportunity to hear the most. When he comes out of the partition within the range of visibility, we pretend not to see him because we do not want to interfere with the doctrine of Gandhism which he heard just now. By the time my turn comes, Mr. Ramapani usually gets too exhausted to spend so much time with me.

I tried to praise his new watch band once to show my appreciation for the finer things in life. Mr. Ramapani sent me back to my files.

For the next few days, we remain disciplined. Absolute examples of ideal workforce. Only the ceiling fans move and make groaning sounds to remind someone that they need oiling. The pages of the calendar flutter with the air. Up and down. Up and down. The fresh page of the new month looks down at us from behind Mr. Basu's head. It reminds us that time flows by.

And since it reminds us that time flows by, we look at our watches. "Teatime!"

And teatimes are teatimes.

Teatimes come no matter which date or which month the calendar shows. It does not interfere with teatimes. For a while, we forget the calendar as we walk towards the canteen to be refreshed.

Teatimes are the times when we leave the files alone to let them air under the fan. Drawers are closed noisily. Chairs are pulled out with dragging ease before we walk our way towards the canteen.

Politics and India's diplomatic relationship with Vietnam is discussed. Share prices, bulls, and bears are explained by Mr. Jha because he studies the market everyday. Mr. Kanjilal discusses the problems he is facing at home because his wife has somehow come to know about his relationship with Ms. Anne, who has joined the office recently as a stenographer.

We finish our tea break with our concern for Mr. Kanjilal and the trouble he is facing at home. We however assure him to follow his heart and to be sure that the rest of the things will follow.

"Poor Kanjilal." We talk to ourselves as we get back inside the office in front of the calendar.

The calendar page flutters in the light breeze of the ceiling fan. The dates of the front page stand in uniform in their respective rows and columns like disciplined boy scouts. The weekdays at the head of each column look at us like troupe leaders.

Seven troupe leaders leading the dates with an equal show of discipline.

I look away.

I look away because I can never get along with so much order. Otherwise instead of joining this office, I could have joined the army. I sincerely consider that too much of order is bad for my health. What if I get hypertension? And what if I get hypertension attacking me with my unfinished files sitting in front of me with all those unfinished calculations? What could happen to all those numbers in the pages of the file, which are, in their highly disorganised order, waiting to get added or subtracted?

I yawn.

I yawn again.

It happens so that they make me yawn again and again.

So I get up to fill some smoke into my lungs so that all the yawns get pushed out in one go.

Talking about yawns reminded me of Mr. Dey, who retired just last year. His chair is now occupied by Wasim Khan.

Mr. Dey would start his yawns when he would be needed to stamp and submit our files, which would go from our table to his.

Once he swallowed something while he was in that process of yawning. We assured him that it certainly could not be a mosquito because it was not yet the rainy season. Mr. Dey was doubtful about that, because he believed that it was none other than female anopheles which he had swallowed, because the female anopheles variety start breeding from the month of June itself.

The calendar page with the month of June flew right in front of his eyes. Mr. Basu had tried to cover the page with his broad back and shoulder when Mr. Dey was showing signs of throwing up.

"What if it was a real female anopheles?"

Mr. Dey drank a lot of water because peon Ravi assured him that mosquitoes cannot bite inside anybody's stomach.

"Even if it did, nothing will happen because your peptides would defend your body." Mr. Basu was more technical in his assurance.

Only when Mr. Dey had drunk enough glasses of water and was convinced that the process of peristalsis was complete did he settle down.

And only after he had settled down did Mr. Basu expose the page of the calendar once again. The month of June thus unveiled had been there for some time, cautioning one and all not to yawn till the rainy season was there, around you and around the office. Hence I am usually careful about yawning, be it February, be it March. However, when I look down into my file with the disorganised numbers and calculations, yawns keep pushing out of my lungs with greater and greater frequency. So there is some need to fill my lungs with smoke.

The calendar watches me go out of the room. It watches over everything.

And everything looks back at it. The month of April stands at the head of the page as the guardian angel. After some days the month of May will lead the troupe.

I will be out and after some time I will be in. A great philosophical concept was taking shape in my mind. Perhaps it showed on my face also. Because Ms. Anne got extremely worried when she saw me staring at the calendar with my face having a Socrates look.

That is why she offered me a glass of water. And because she had offered me a glass of water, I continued to look very sick.

How sick you are depends on who is nursing you.

But there certainly was some misunderstanding because of Ms. Anne offering me a glass of water. Mr. Kanjilal did not like the move. A harmless move of a pretty Ms. Anne offering me, her sick colleague, a glass of water.

To show how disappointed he was with us, he did not come to the canteen with us to have tea. And when we offered him our invitation, he gave the excuse that he had those files to clear and that he came to the office strictly to work and not waste his time like us. He also said something else, which nobody could hear because he muttered it very softly, perhaps with his teeth joined together.

So he stayed back with the calendar.

And he stayed back with his work and the calendar. He thus stayed back for two more days and he continued his sulking. This gave Mr. Wasim Khan the wrong impression.

So on the day after that, we saw him gazing at the calendar. He had the same Socrates look. However this time, before Ms. Anne could offer him the glass of water, we found that Mr. Kanjilal was already there with his glass of water.

And since it was Mr. Kanjilal who was nursing the "calendar attacked" Mr. Wasim Khan, and not pretty Ms. Anne, as was expected by everybody, the sickness was gone with just a glass of water.

There was no question of dragging out the attack, because Mr. Kanjilal was glaring at Mr. Wasim Khan with his fierce look.

Mr. Basu tried to have the calendar attack when Mr. Kanjilal was on leave. And because Ms. Anne voluntarily took up the task of nursing Mr. Basu, no one in the office had anything to say. We knew that Mr. Basu was in safe hands. And Mr. Basu also knew that he was in safe hands.

So he tried to lean all his weight on Ms. Anne.

Ms. Anne, for her part, rested him back on his chair. Mr. Basu had to turn back to look at the calendar and get the "calendar attack." The space between his table and his chair was not enough for him to turn back to his position that easily, without Ms. Anne's help, as he had got stuck in between.

Everything went on smoothly that day because Mr. Kanjilal was on leave. So there was no misunderstanding.

The calendar remained there on the wall, letting its pages fly like proud banners. Proud banners of time.

The calendar makes us wait for the Salary Day at the end of every month. The most welcome date.

"Would you push your head sideways, Mr. Basu? Let me count the number of days between today and the salary day." Mr. Ratan Pathak wants to make sure.

"Which day of the week is the next government holiday?" I ask Mr. Basu to look back and tell us.

And Mr. Basu turns to look at the calendar.

My question is answered. "Next holiday is a Monday."

My problem is solved by Mr. Basu.

But Mr. Basu has created his problem.

He has got stuck, once again, between his chair and his table. We wait for Ms. Anne to help him back to position.

The Field

One day I will be living in the still world of a group home, when Mother won't be around to take care of me anymore. I may spend my time in a room, watching a field, imagining Emma to be around somewhere. I do not know an Emma in real life. Yet I exactly know who she is. And Emma continues to fill my moments of loneliness.

One

How many trees can that field hold? Perhaps a hundred. If all that grass were not there and if someone cared to plant some trees in that place, there could be a whole new way to look at that space.

Someone once asked me why I stare at the stretch of that field so much. I did not see who it was that asked me. Perhaps Jane or perhaps Susan. Surely it was not Emma. Because Emma tells me that she cannot come at certain times, when there are so many voices around me. She can come only when the world around, including the sky, including the walls and that field where I fix my gaze, turns purple mixed with black. She can come only when all other voices go beyond my range of hearing.

When the distant field spreads a thin layer of mist all around itself, and when through the mist you can see or almost see shapes rising up or moving down, and when you can hear or almost hear nothing, not even the sound of footsteps outside, not even the whisper of the air, and when you forget to hear the sound of the clock, you can hear Emma.

Emma never asks anything.

She just knows.

She just knows that the next shadow that would rise up from that mist above the field would go towards that distant factory chimney, which seems to float in the sea of fog.

Emma just knows that the shapes forming and dissolving in the mist never want anyone to actually know anything about them. They just happen to want to be whatever they are. Emma tells me how difficult it really is to be what you are. Everyone seems to want to be something else other than what he really is.

She never asks.

She just knows.

The field was now filled with a nine o'clock morning sunshine. I wonder how it would look with trees instead of that grass-covered stretch. And how many trees could that field actually hold? Emma should know.

She just knows.

Two

It was just a hat. His Sunday hat, as they were telling each other. And everything about their talk went in and out around his Sunday hat.

Someone dropped a cup of tea accidentally inside it while watching a game show on the television. I could hear his voice screaming at the tea and game lover. It was his angry voice. He usually has this angry voice when he comes here in the mornings to take his rounds. He peeps inside every room and gets disgusted to see so much mess around all over. He is sure that nothing ever will be better, even if Mr. Beck comes sooner than he is supposed to.

I think Mr. Beck would replace him in a few weeks. That's what those voices tell each other. All those voices outside my door speak in a very low tone whenever he is around. They do not laugh. And they do not talk much to each other.

I wonder about Mr. Beck.

Does he wear a hat too on Sundays? A black Sunday hat?

I heard them coming towards my door. As they came near, their speech got louder and slowly moved further and further away, to blend with all those noises of the world.

I thought about hats. A world full of hats. Lots of black Sunday hats with lots of tea spilling over them.

How would that field look like if all those Sunday hats covered all that green grass on it?

Only Emma would know how it would look.

She just knows.

Emma would never come here in this noise. But she will come for sure. When all that noise around gets quiet or almost quiet, when the world turns purple mixed with black and when you can see your shadow in the whole world, you can hear Emma coming. You do not need to see Emma. You just know she is there. And, only if you are hearing carefully, you can hear her voice.

Emma never wants you to be distracted by any other sound. She says nothing if you are hearing those paper bits flying around in front of your table fan. She would not go away but she would surely stop. And even if you wished that she spoke, she just would not.

I think she could come in a hat this time. A black Sunday hat.

But I needed to wait. I waited with my thoughts filled with hats. A world full of hats. Lots of black Sunday hats.

Three

A bigger head would have done more justice to him. It was rather too small compared to his great size and his big brown shoes. I carefully saw the window reflect in his shoes as he turned and pointed them towards it.

I was impressed.

I next wanted to see that tree, which was behind the window, reflect in it. I had to wait for him to turn and walk a little further towards the window.

I waited. And I waited.

He did nothing to move towards that window. They always neglect to see so many things. And they miss out on so much.

For instance, they hardly seem to notice the shadow of the nail on that wall outside on the yard. The sun makes it shift all along through the day. It follows the order of the sun. They hardly notice. Emma tells me that they see it all. But they have so many things to look at that they do not bother to really think about it as I do. "Does it matter anyway?" she had asked me once. "Does it matter anyway," I had to tell her back.

Some days I become like the mirror and I need to tell back all that is being told to me. It does not matter what is being told. As long as it is being told. Does it matter to the mirror anyway what object is in front of it? It reflects the object anyway.

Emma understands my "mirror days." But many people don't. Usually people who are new here or are visiting this place do wonder why I talk back all those words which they say. They wonder for a while and then they get used to it.

I had to get used to his small head anyway. But I needed to wait to see the reflection of that tree behind the window in his shining brown shoes.

I waited. And I waited.

But I could no longer wait. I just needed to do something to see the reflection of the tree behind the window in his shining brown shoes. What if he went away? And what if I never saw the reflection anymore? Certainly I could not push the tree near his shoes. But I could always push him towards the window. Obviously they had to move me away from him. Perhaps I cried. Perhaps I screamed. I do not remember.

When Emma comes next, I will surely know.

Emma should know.

She just knows.

Four

How fast can that ant crawl?

The ant took its time to climb up the tabletop to find some sugar grains, which were lying there since I had my tea.

They give me tea in the evening. Every evening. That is what they were told from the very beginning.

There is a very beginning of everything.

Very beginning of a story, very beginning of a movie, very beginning of the road, very beginning of a task, and very beginning of all those things that have ends.

Emma tells me that there are certain things that have no end. For example time. It was always there and there is no end to it. She is certain that even when there was absolutely nothing around, even when there was no such thing as that field or evening tea, there was time.

She knows it all.

She just knows.

And from the very beginning they gave me tea at this hour of evening. Who told them to do so? I do not remember at all. Perhaps I was never sure which beginning I needed to remember. I had many beginnings. Beginning of the end of my school, beginning of the death of Mother and learning to live without her, beginning of my many new homes, beginning of my living inside a mirror and not knowing how to come out, and beginning of the feeling of Emma with me.

She will not be with me now.

When the world turns purple mixed with black and when all the shadows mix up with my own shadow, when you can hear or almost hear nothing, Emma is with me. Did she have a beginning?

The ant was patient with time. It was in no hurry. It slowly went from one corner of the tablecloth and picked up the sugar grain. There were more grains around. But it just held on to one. Did it get confused about which sugar grain it should choose to pick? Or did it not matter at all to the ant whether it made the right choice?

I will never know.

But I knew for sure that it would come back with others to collect the rest of the sugar grains.

Last week, when I needed to become a stairway and when Sam tried to move me from his way to the kitchen and found my body too heavy to be lifted up, he had to come back with others to remove me from the way. There was a difference. The difference was that Sam had to hurry, and could not be patient like the ant.

The ant crawled down the table now. I needed to wait for it to come back. Alone or with others. I needed to be patient.

All that time, which had no beginning and no end, recorded my patience within it.

Five

The glass of water stood still on the table. There was a sort of absoluteness in it. Only an extreme peace can bring that sort of absoluteness in any thing. There seemed to be no difference between this glass of water and a rock.

It reflected the tree right behind the window. I saw those little leaves move slightly in their reflection. Like a little stray thought in the stillness.

Like a thought of Emma in the stillness around. The thought of Emma never disturbs any peace. It is always a part of it.

The field covered with grass lay stretched in the sunlight. It got filled up with all her thoughts. There was no turbulence anywhere. All her thoughts extended from there to the air that was dense with morning chill.

Yet it remained peaceful. There was no wind.

Emma's thoughts were spreading all around. It touched me.

Someone was calling me. I did not move. Any movement would upset the absoluteness around.

Someone called me louder. And then louder again.

His voice cut through the absoluteness like a saw. It created a divide in the air, in the surface of water, in its reflections, and in that field. His voice divided the absoluteness into two parts. One part had all the thoughts of Emma. The other part had his voice.

My senses got ripped off. A few remained on the other side with thoughts of Emma. The rest shifted to the side of his voice. Each side tried to complete itself by closing the torn part.

I saw the front growing turbulent.

There was no use of that glass of water anymore. I dropped all that water around, scattering the glass pieces everywhere.

Six

The cloud had come from the eastern corner to almost settle its shadow over the field. Then came the next cloud and then another. They all competed with each other to settle their shadow over that field.

However, they happened to form a truce between themselves. They joined together. They joined together, to fill up the whole sky, and settled right upon the earth.

A strange light filled the spaces around. It was neither too dark nor too bright. It was green.

I knew that the green light came from the trees and that field. Emma should have seen it. But she would not be able to come now. She can come only when everything around turns dark or almost dark, when all the world around looks like a big black field to the stars, and when you can hear or almost hear nothing but quietness. I am sure she knows about the green light, which comes out from the trees and that field, after the clouds settle upon the earth.

Emma just knows.

Now the wind started to blow. They usually send someone to keep an eye over me when the wind starts blowing rough. Ever since I ran out of the gate believing myself to be the wind, they send someone with some tea into my room.

It makes my work very difficult. For I have to choose between being the wind or drinking the cup of tea. I cannot experience the wind and the tea together. I knew someone would come any moment inside my room and fill up all the space with his presence.

It will be like those clouds filling up the spaces in the sky. I wondered what colour I would see around me. Certainly it would not remain green anymore. Perhaps the colour of tea.

Seven

No one knew from where it came. Yet no one wanted to find out. Because every one wanted it to stay here with us.

Someone began to call it Tom. And Tom seemed to like that name. So it would look up each time someone called it Tom. It would even expect someone to throw a biscuit at it as a reward.

I would wonder about its former home. Did it have any memories about its former master? Or was it a homeless nameless dog? Free from any name, like that big rock outside the gate where David and Carlos sit to smoke.

I think that rock would love to have some name. Emma tells me "No." She thinks that rocks and dust grains that fill up the whole world do not want to be tied up to any kind of home and name. Homes and names bind you to them. Rocks and dust grains do not like any form of bondage. They know that bondages bring concerns. And concerns take away all that peace to which they owe their very presence.

That is why they do not cry or scream when they are pushed from one position to another. They can be anywhere on the face of earth. Call them this or call them that.

I saw Tom play with others through the window.

I can never play. And how could I really play with anyone when I have to remind myself in so many ways that I am supposed to be playing and not staring at my shadow wondering about its length during teatime? So I never play. I never play because I cannot play.

Emma tells me that I need not have to do everything that most others can do. "It really is important what you are and think and less important as to what you can do."

Emma knows it all. She just knows.

Tom would love her, I am sure. But Emma hardly lets anyone know that she is there. And what if Tom became noisy after seeing her? Emma cannot be there when there is any noise around. She can only come when all the noise around stops and when you can hear or almost hear nothing.

I could hear them play. I could hear them call Tom from all around the courtyard.

And then I could hear nothing.

I could think about nothing, but Emma.

Eight

The bird was making a great deal of noise.

My mother used to tell me that it was a good sign. Birds make noise because they know from the beginning that you may have guests.

"And how do they know?"

"Simple," she would say. "When they fly, they can see much more than we do.

"They can see the whole length of the road. So if anyone came this way, they would know. It would not miss their eyes."

I never wanted guests. I never trusted them. They would come and they would talk. They would talk about their happiness, their homes, and their children. And how well their wonderful children were doing in their schools. Every child was destined to be great men and women.

Once, one of them brought her son with her. He was my age.

He could do all those things which I could not. He could ask my mother why I never spoke anything. Once satisfied that I could not, he came near me and spoke in my ears several times, "You are a donkey."

"What are you telling him?" his mother wanted to know.

"I am telling him a fun story."

How old was I then? And what did I do? I had asked Emma. She told me, "It does not matter." Emma tells me it should not matter at all. I want to believe her. I always believe her. And why shouldn't I?

Emma just knows.

Mother had nothing to talk to those guests. She would listen and cook them a meal. She would just let them talk and then, when they finished their talk, she would let them go.

We would not hear the noise of any bird after they left.

I heard the bird calling out. I know there would be no visitors today. Visitors are supposed to come here only on Sundays. I do not have any visitor. How would I have? Ever since the death of Mother, ever since I began to live either outside the mirror or inside the mirror, and ever since Emma came to me, I stopped expecting guests. And very few people here have guests. Only those who are meant to be forgotten stay here. That is what Emma thinks.

"It does not matter.

"And it should not matter." She is never wrong.

Who knows what that bird could see?

Nine

The field lay with its grass and little pebbles. It lay stretching in the sunshine. It lay stretching below the sun, wishing that it was cooled by a shade of a cloud. Yet it kept its wish all to itself. There was no complaint.

Emma tells me that when a wish grows bigger, it becomes an expectation. Expectation is always in a hurry to be fulfilled. So it gets impatient and begins to complain.

The field is in no hurry. It has seen the beginning of the earth. It has seen the beginning and end of many lives around it. Perhaps it saw the rise and fall of many civilizations and kingdoms. Its measure of time is very different from what the clock tells us.

So it can only wish. And that is what it does all day and through the night. It wishes to grow and fill the whole world and embrace it all around. Sometimes it wishes to grow a flower garden in it. Sometimes it wishes to have a whole colony of anthills on its stretch, with little ants crawling all around it, tickling its body.

Sometimes it wonders what others think about it. Does

it know that the full moon always wishes to be rolled on its stretch?

Does it know that I want to plant a forest on it?

And does it know that whenever I stare at it, they ask me what I look at so much, out over there?

How many trees can it really hold? Perhaps a hundred. I should not forget to ask Emma. She would surely know.

She just knows.

The Climb

Salvador Dalí always inspires me. In fact, most of his surreal paintings compel me to try and put words into some similar dream situation — climbing into a dream, following the promises of clouds. I followed my story around the hill towards some unknown dream.

The Climb

Steeper and higher became the climb as I tried to hurry my steps on the slope. The sun, which was behind me all along until now, suddenly seemed to hurry ahead of me, showing the evening glow.

The rock goats which scattered here and there like those scattered stones and pebbles totally ignored my presence. I ignored them too. For I needed to reach the other side of the hill before it got dark.

And what should I do when I reached the other side? Well, I had to find out first what the other side looked like. Only then would I know what to do.

I did not choose any road this time. Because roads did restrict your steps in one direction. And when you see other passersby taking the same route, you realize that you are only following them.

Yet everything followed everything. Summer followed winter. Day followed night, pretty moon followed the earth. And in the cycle of human life, old age followed the strength of youthfulness, while death followed everything. Nature too had plenty of rules to follow. Those rock goats there had some grass and weeds to follow. And I followed my dream.

My dream followed nothing.

I walked and I climbed as the evening sun was drowning down below my sight. Soon the night would cover everything, making the climbing almost impossible. I looked back. I could not see any road down there. There was no reason now to go back and follow any road, after climbing till here.

And I realized that I was also following something, though it was not any road. I was left hanging on the hill while the sun was climbing down, while the rock goats were climbing down, and while the night was descending upon the earth.

I was still climbing up. I was seeking something to sit on for the night. Rest followed.

The Rest

And sure and stealthy came the night
On the sky and in my sight

The hill and heavens side by side
Lay around me in the quiet.

Was the wind blowing? I think so. For I could smell the wildflowers, which were not nearby, as I looked around me. I sat on
a big black rock waiting to get used to the darkness. I needed
to go to the other side of the hill.

And whatever be there on the other side
May be new to me
For the sky had promised me
My road to dream there shall be.

And my dream was as impossible as the purple sun and orange
clouds. It was as impossible as glass-winged blue butterflies
flying under that purple sun and those orange clouds. The sky
had promised me that it was there. All I needed to do was follow the morning star during the early dawn and the little boat-
shaped cloud during the later mornings.

I could not afford to miss the cloud shaped like a boat.
Because the cloud never waited for anybody, let alone me.
Why should it? It had to travel the whole of the earth, showing dreamers like me how to reach their dreams. So if I
missed it by chance, I had to wait for a complete day for its
return.

And thus I followed all my day
The cloud leading me all my way
Till I reached this lonely hill
And sat the dark hours in the still.

And now as I sat on the big black rock waiting for the night to glide through the surroundings, smelling some wildflowers, I felt a soft touch on my knee.

It was a rock goat.

Rock Goat

"It has lost its way," I thought at first. It sat close to me with its eyes shining in the darkness. And then it insisted me to follow it, through its own way of communication. It gently began to push on my knees with its head.

And I followed it. Sometimes towards the other side of the hill and sometimes upwards on the hill where the stones got bigger and bigger. I was not used to these hilly tracks, and so I was very careful as I followed the rock goat.

I crawled and I slipped
And misplaced my feet
I was clumsy I admit
But I would not accept any defeat.

Bushes appeared on the way. And bushes disappeared behind our way. The rock goat was very patient with me. It gave me time to adjust my steps on the uneven track, waiting here and waiting there. Proceeding now and waiting then. I did not ask it to wait when I was trying to balance on one of those angularly edged rocks. I just knew that it would wait.

We crossed the bushes and we crossed the bends.

The beginning of a rock and an abrupt end.

As I paused to take my breaths, I could see the moon rising in the sky through some distant mist. And I could see the distant mist trying to rise with it, as if regretting letting it go. I saw the strange communication of the moon, the mist, the sky, and the earth. The rock goat nudged me with its head, only to remind me that I needed to follow it.

> The night seemed long
> The mist was on
> The earth and sky in spread
> As the night
> In moon light
> Looked ghostly as the dead.

Time seemed to be eternal as I followed the rock goat. The hill seemed to grow bigger and stretch wider as the night continued with my footsteps. Nothing seemed to look familiar after a while. The colour of the rocks and stones changed into lighter colours of grey. I now turned back only to see the distant sky turning bright. I realized that I had lost my way. The rock goat had also disappeared somewhere, leaving me on some nowhere of the hill from where the big black rock on which I had sat last evening could not be seen.

I had to find it first because the boat-shaped cloud would lead me from there to my dream, which was as impossible as the land where glass-winged blue butterflies flew under the purple sun and orange clouds.

Hermit of the Hill

"Many many years ago, when the sky and the earth touched each other on this hill, when rock goats went to the other side, which was lit up by the first rays of the sun, to dance around the talking weeds all morning, till the shadow of rocks grew small under the midday sun, there lived a solitary hermit in a cave that is lost with time.

"And all through the day, he sat on that big black rock trying to listen to what those rock goats sang about. And surely those rock goats sang about the world below the hill from where they came. A busy busy world. And a noisy cheerful world."

The world from which they came
Was not any same
Like this solitary mountain.

"And every day the rock goats would tell each other the wonderful stories of a fair maiden who lived down in the village just below the hill. The stones would hear it. The weeds would hear it. And the hermit would hear it.

"'She dances the best
With her fair footsteps
Charming the hearts,
With her cheer and grace.'

"The hermit forgot about his meditation. He forgot about the peaceful hill which was beyond the joys and sorrows of those busy villages. And the rock goats promised to lead him there.

"So one evening, when the sun was setting behind a growing mist, he followed those rock goats."

He must have faltered,
He must have climbed,
He must have given up
At some point of time.

"He could not complain that the sky had not warned him. He could not complain that the big rock did not warn him. Everyone told him that the rock goats would not lead him anywhere. 'You say so because you want me to stay trapped in peace like you.' He was heard for the last time. Nobody argued anymore. Because Nature warns but never argues. The hermit began to follow the rock goats before disappearing out of sight."

And the mist approached
With stealthy float
Covering the hill and earth
The hermit of
The lonely hill
Was never seen of or heard.

And the sky breathed a heavy sigh with the West Wind.

"Did he reach the village? Did he meet the fair maiden?" I asked.

The sky became silent. I tried to reach the big black rock from where the rock goat had led me into the lost nothingness of the hill. I needed to reach it before the boat-shaped cloud appeared. For it would lead me to my impossible dream, which was as impossible as the glass-winged blue butterflies flying under the purple sun and orange clouds.

The West Wind began to blow stronger.

West Wind

"Did you see that grey rock to your right?"

I had turned around. There was not only one grey rock. I saw many grey rocks planted on the face of the hill. Which rock was the sky showing me?

I did not interrupt, as the view of the sky was much different from my view. My view was limited to that rock and this stone or perhaps that dry bush. The sky had a wider view, and perhaps it meant some rock which was beyond my sight.

Grey stones lay all along my side, left and right, as the sky became blue once again. And just as the rock goat had disappeared, one by one the stars began to disappear from my sight. The new day was wiping out every trace of night. And since I could not identify the grey stone which the sky was trying to show me, I took for granted that it was the biggest one with a smooth surface which the sky meant.

"That is where Adam's grave is."

Old as he was
Looking up at the sky
He could wish nothing else
But to die.
For his life on earth
Was hard and cursed

His bones had grown old
He was breathing his last.

The sky told me how the midday sun had burnt his wrinkled skin, which had folded into complicated furrows with age. How a vulture had waited patiently on a nearby rock, giving him enough time to breathe till his last.

And then the West Wind had blown for the first time on the earth, carrying Adam's last breath with it to the other parts of the world. And then with the West Wind blew the sand and dust which covered the body of Adam right by the edge of that grey stone.

"What about the vulture?" I had asked.

"The vulture was chased away by the wind itself." The sky heaved a sigh which was none other than the West Wind.

I just knew that it carried Adam's last breath with it. I looked for a final time at the big smooth stone. Adam's grave.

But I could not afford to wait. Because I had to find the big black rock from where the boat-shaped cloud would lead me to my dream, which was as impossible as glass-winged blue butterflies flying under a purple sun and orange clouds.

And I followed the wind, which led me to a little clearing.

The Clearing

> The sun looked like a crimson ball.
> Then it turned to gold
> The clouds turned brighter white
> With the day's unfold.

The mist disappeared with it. I could see clearly now everything that the altitude showed me. I was not at the top of the hill. I was somewhere in the middle, with a little flat field in front of me. I could see more hills around me. Except for this flat field, everything looked the same. Some stones, some weeds, some wildflowers belonging to those weeds, and some dry bushes. The everythings coloured with some green here and some brown there. And of course a lot of grey patches here and there.

And I waited for all that my eyes could show me in the hope to see a glimpse of something black. I was sure that it could be none other than the big black rock where I had sat before the rock goat brought me in this nowhere zone of the hill. And if only I found it, I could be sure to see the boat-shaped cloud which would lead me to my dream, which was as impossible as the glass-winged blue butterflies flying under a purple sun and orange clouds.

*   *   *

There was no point in asking the sky. The view of the sky was wider than my view. It had the unlimited stretch of vastness which could not be judged with my petty limits.

"There on the hill where the weeds did not grow,
The Sun God had landed his chariot once, long long ago."

I knew the sky was talking about the clearing on which I stood.

"When the great flood had drowned the earth, including the hill, and the rains had poured and poured to show how much they could pour, and when the animals had looked with greater fear at the stretch of water which had covered the earth around the Ark, the Sun God took pity on them and decided to dry the earth for those poor lives.

"So after the rains stopped, the earth was trying to dry up. Because the rains had caused such a swamp that it was impossible to step down from the Ark. The animals got their feet buried in that swamp.

"It was then that the Sun God felt pity on those poor animals. He stood there on that place with his flaming chariot drying up the earth, till the ground got drier and harder.

"Sun God had climbed back to the sky.
The earth on the hill became very dry.

The animals on the earth thrived and thrived
Since that flood of the age gone by.

"However, the place where the Sun God had landed had become so hot that grasses and weeds refused to grow there."

I touched the dry clearing. I could not feel any heat. But I knew that it was warm because the sky told me that it was warm. And the weeds knew that it was warm.

Wildflowers

Wildflowers are plenty on the earth. Yet I never even took any notice of them until I came here. Only on the bend of the hill did I see those wildflowers, the smell of which was reaching me time and again as the wind blew.

I should not say "bend of the hill" because the hill by its structure was nothing but bend. So the bend was more related to my footsteps and my direction. When I stood on the lonely hill, the world seemed to exist all around me, and I related everything to my perceptions. Like how it becomes a hot day when you feel hot. And it becomes a dull day when you are bored. So on that slope, I felt that the sky and earth kept me as the centre. Again those distant eagles that encircled a piece of sky out over there seemed to be related to the piece of sky over my head.

And now when I was so close to those wildflowers, smelling their wild smells, I wondered what their names could be. Again, everything on the earth need not be named or be familiar to you. If that was so, then every other flower could be called a hibiscus or a rose.

The flowers intoxicated me with their scents.

> Maybe it was because of my sleepless night
> Or maybe because of their pretty sight
> Maybe because of some other "why"
> Sleep came down, on my blessed eyes.

Perhaps the sun had warned me with the midday heat. Perhaps the wind had shouted aloud into my ears. Perhaps the sky had told me a secret story about those wildflowers. I cannot say anything about them. Because I was fast asleep with those flowers around me.

How long did I sleep? I think for hours. Because when I awoke, the sun had already turned orange. And I chose to go left. There was no reason to go left whatsoever. As if any direction mattered in a lost path. The sky was anywhere around on my left or on my right making no difference.

The sky was silent when I accused it for my sleep. For I knew that I was delayed by hours.

Wildflowers nodded and swayed
A pretty sight yes they made
Filling my heart profound
With the wind blowing around.

Soon the sun got out of sight.

The flowers too were out of sight.

Only my dream remained, which was as impossible as glass-winged blue butterflies flying under a purple sun and orange clouds.

Again the Night

"A full moon has many secrets. Those which it will not reveal," the sky complained. "And the earth loves it because of that.

"And the blue star right over your head loves it because of that.

"And perhaps the rising mist loves it because of that."

I saw the rising mist. It had its own secrets. And as it surrounded everything with its enchanting embrace, I saw everything becoming a part of its secret. Then it became a big guess as I wondered what lay hidden in it. The smoking cold mist was rising with the moon. I waited. And I waited, because I had nothing else to do.

Everything which the daylight had shown me looked different in the darkness and the smoking mist. The hill itself looked like an outlined black smoke. And how did I look standing there on that hill slope?

There was no rock goat anywhere to move the stillness around. And the wait looked long. As if everything around waited for some movement. And those rocks which were planted on the face or back of the hill had a longer wait. Their waiting was determined by nature since God knows when. Perhaps that rock over there waited to be shifted from there to here.

"And why not shift that rock from there to here?" After all, I needed to spend the time. And I could also end some long wait which would contribute to changing something on the face of the earth. So I started to dig.

The rock was planted deeper than what I had thought. The ground was also reluctant to give it up that easily. And as usual, Nature resisted. Nature refuses anyone to upset its order. And I was trying to reshape it by digging the rock from there and planning to plant it here.

> The rock was big
> For me to dig
> Yet I carried on
> I heard it sound
> On the ground

I persisted all along.
And night stood still
On the hill
The moon climbed up and up
It had a smile
Of a secret style
It watched my worthless work.

I looked at the hollow I had made after removing the rock. It looked back at me with that single eye like a haunting eye. I looked away as I tried to plant the rock not here, but some distance away.

The moon and the mist gathered around it as some secret. Was I included in that secret?

Staring Hole

And secrets lay all around
The land and in the air
All of it stared at me
With some secret stare.

As the air around me grew into a breeze, and then into a wind, as the moon allowed itself to get tossed from one cloud to the next, hiding now and revealing then, I tried to cover up the hole which I had dug when I removed the rock. I put some pebbles and some earth into it. For the hole looked at me with hollowness of a staring eye. As if it asked some secret question.

And that secret question could be anything. Anything like "What should I look at?" or "Whose eye am I?" or "Why can't I close my eyelids?" Secret questions needed a lot of guessing to answer. So you either ignore them or you try to stop them. I could not ignore them. So I tried to stop them.

> In a way, I may say
> All those quests on earth,
> Need not be told aloud,
> And need not be heard.

So I tried to fill the hole up and stop those questions. First I collected some loose stones which were lying here and there. Then I gathered dust and weeds. Everything went into it. But the eye remained. So I dug out more holes and transferred their earth into it.

And in that busy process, I forgot about the big black rock which I had to find. I forgot about the morning star and the boat-shaped cloud which would lead me to my impossible dream. And then I forgot about my dream, which was as impossible as glass-winged blue butterflies flying under a purple sun and orange clouds.

> And thus the night had passed away
> As the darkness dawned
> The moon too had faded out
> With a bright new morn.

I realized that my last drop of water was gone when the last pebble got into the hole, filling it to my satisfaction. I felt a great thirst rising within me.

I needed to search for water before continuing my search for the big black rock. Water was more necessary at that moment. And dream was a fancy. And dreams could wait.

Water

Surely water could be found somewhere around in the hill. And why shouldn't it be found? The hill was big enough for anything. And I was not asking the sky to lead me to a camel or a whale. All I wanted it to tell me was how to find water. And water was not an impossible dream.

"Look to your west on the further end of the slope downhill. And look around for the Talking Stone. You may find water. Because the Stone will tell you where water is."

The sky fell silent once again.
I needed to act fast
As my throat felt the thirst.
The morning spread to light my way
And again came another day.

And I found the Talking Stone as I accidentally stepped on it. The moment I heard it groan, I knew that it could be none other than the Talking Stone. The Stone would not tell me the way to water unless I told it the secret of the tree which never had its shadow.

Why the hell did it want to know? I could not ask it. It obviously had some reason I suppose. Whatever be the reason, I needed to find the tree without any shadow. Only then would I be able to find water.

And I knew very well that without water I would not be able to search the big black rock from where the rock goat had led me to some lost nowhere of the hill. And without the big black rock I would not be able to follow the boat-shaped cloud which would lead me to my dream, which was as impossible as glass-winged butterflies flying under a purple sun and orange clouds.

Finding any tree on the rocky hill was not easy. Let alone a tree without a shadow. Yet for the sake of my thirst I was prepared to do that.

I could either go up or I could go down. I decided to go down.

> Down the slope I hurried my way
> For some impossible tree
> All my eyes had to say
> Stones and weeds it could see.

> Yes it was a search
> And lengthy search it was
> Then as if through Heaven's grace
> The sound of a stream I heard.

And at that moment I thought that I had found a very precious dream. More precious than any impossible dream.

> Water!
> I touched it, I drank it,
> I poured it over my head
> And then with an aching tiredness
> By the stream I slept.

Did the boat-shaped cloud come and go? I was not bothered. I was just tired. Very tired.

> And I heard the flowing stream
> Even in my dream.

And limitless impossibility with its limitless search was waiting as I slept.

Limitless Search

The sky does not know the meaning of limit. And can never comprehend the meaning of boundary. As I was already by the stream, I did not really need to go back to the Talking Stone. Nor did I need to find any tree which had no shadow. I had my boundary of patience which was again bounded by time. And all those boundaries were for some unbounded dream of mine which was as impossible as glass-winged blue butterflies flying under a purple sun and orange clouds.

The sky reminded me that the Talking Stone was waiting for me. And I argued that I did not require its help. The sky pointed out that the Talking Stone had been waiting for me. And its wait was longer than my wait. I faced the stream.

And I saw the sun reflect in it. When everything around on the hill was still, the sight of the moving water was so welcoming to my eyes that I was prepared to see the running water instead of my dream. And I saw the sky reflect in the stream. I heard the reminder from its reflection. I knew that I had to go.

I had to go from this place to that where there was a tree which had no shadow just because there was a Talking Stone which was waiting for me. The thoughts of mine kept company with my reluctant steps. The sky watched over.

Sometimes my thoughts flowed towards the Talking Stone, and sometimes, whenever the West Wind blew, they flowed towards Adam's grave. Thoughts could flow in any direction. But I had to choose some direction to follow, as there was no road to lead me.

> I crossed the stream and I crossed some weeds and grass.
> I crossed the staring rocks and crossed the this and thats.
> I climbed sometimes upwards and then went downwards.
> And when the sun had glided west, a tree I observed.

But when I reached the tree, the sun had already gone out of sight. All I was left to do now was to wait. The greater shadow of the night merged with a bigger shadow spreading across the earth.

The limitless sky merged with that shadow. I was part of it.

And Continued Wait

Every wait need not be idle. And every idle moment need not be a static one. Although the darkness was posing to show

how idle it was, I knew it was not idle. In fact, it looked busier than any day. For all those dreams and all those thoughts moved around everything near and far. They were touching all those known corners of the stream, the Talking Stone and Adam's grave, from where the West Wind was blowing. And they also touched the sun and the daylight on the far away other side of the world, the same way as they touched my dream beyond the world, which was as impossible as glass-winged blue butterflies flying under a purple sun and orange clouds.

The sky had a cloudy veil. The moon looked like a blurred patch of white with a diffused edge. With its faint light, it could not create any shadow under anything. I looked at the moon because there was nothing else to look at. I lay on my back looking at it, as motionless as those stones and the tree which could be the tree without any shadow. I was one of those stones with my motionless wait.

> And the night was high on sky
> And the night was low on earth
> And the night with west wind blew
> To the elsewheres to continue ...

And the night continued with the traveling moon. It continued with a silver snake which was traveling through its familiar track towards the tree. It continued with the snake's cold ripples as it climbed over my left leg and travelled down again into some other "again" and some other "after that." For every "after that" has another "after that" to continue.

I could have jumped out of fear when the snake was crossing my leg. Strangely, I did not. I realized what a powerful influence the idle stones had on me. Time passed from some instant to some other instant.

Yet the wait continued all through those instants. Somewhere the Talking Stone waited. The secret of the tree without a shadow waited to be revealed. Night waited. And I waited.

Of course every possible or impossible dream waited.

Rolling Stone

While everything waited with some patience and some restlessness, with some stillness and some movement along with me, I saw it roll slowly uphill. And what else could move like that other than a Rolling Stone?

The little stone moved uphill, defying every rule of gravity. And I was definitely not dreaming. It slowly climbed up, tempting me with every impossibility of itself to follow it. "Should I lose sight of the tree? Should I follow the Rolling Stone?" The secret of the tree without any shadow could wait and the Talking Stone's quest could wait. But a Rolling Stone would not wait. I climbed the rock just above the tree to follow the Rolling Stone. The Rolling Stone speeded up.

The Rolling Stone climbed up a rock above the tree.

The rock was big, and I found it quite an effort to climb on it. When I finally climbed up on it, I could see that the rock was peeping down. It peeped down to the treetop and it peeped down to the place where I was lying down. Rolling Stone waited for me on the peeping rock. When I was ready, it began to move ahead, leading me to God knows where. And one follow led to another. I was getting used to all of it.

> And all those things that are on earth
> May not be earthly enough
> As are truths that fill the heart
> As some heavenly love.

And so was the impossibility of the Rolling Stone moving uphill, so was the impossibility of the quest of the Talking Stone. My impossible dream got closer to me.

The eastern sky showed a faint glow, reminding me about the tree which did not have any shadow. I had to watch over it. I had to tell the Talking Stone what I had watched. I had to find the big black rock where I had sat before following the rock goat. And I had to follow a boat-shaped cloud which would lead me to my dream, which was as impossible as glass-winged blue butterflies flying under a purple sun and orange clouds.

The Rolling Stone stopped rolling as I got obsessed with my thoughts. And it continued to be still even when I moved closer, leaving me in a fix as to whether it moved at all or not. It looked like any other stone which lay all around. Qualities lie hidden.

Daylight was showing everything. Soon the sun would be seen. I hurried towards the peeping rock, under which the tree waited with some secret.

The King and the Rolling Stone

> "And the Rolling Stone you saw
> Is one and only found
> For no stone could roll as pleased
> On the hill or ground."

I continued to rest myself on the peeping stone from where I could watch over the tree which did not have any shadow. I did not look back even when the sky told me that the Rolling Stone was unique. The sun was now turning orange and then gold. My eyes concentrated under the tree.

"And the king who ruled this hill
Owned the yonder arounds
Who by chance had come across
The stone rolling on the ground

"The king was surprised when he saw
The stone rolling up high,
He began to follow the blessed stone
Under the blessed sky.

"Yes the years passed one by one
For seasons changed along
Yet the king followed the stone
In sunshine and in storm."

The sky stopped as suddenly as it started. The sun continued
to climb. I continued to keep an eye under the tree lying on my
chest on the peeping rock. And the peeping rock continued to
peep down at something which I did not know.

The sky continued . . .

"The king had turned old and old
He forgot his kingdom and his gold
For the stone which rolled and rolled
Within his reach but beyond his hold."

"And did he finally get hold of it?" I asked the sky without
looking up.

"Dreams are followed
Dreams are searched
But holding a dream
Is unheard."

The sky stopped with a sigh of the West Wind which brought Adam's last breath with it. I found the king's breaths too in it. I breathed in everything.

Shadowless Tree

While I was still in my early-day idleness, lying on the peeping rock, peeping at the tree down there and breathing in the West Wind, I began to feel sleepy. But I was careful not to sleep because that would delay me further.

And if I was delayed again, I could get trapped into something else and further flow the dream of mine away into the postponement of the yets. I felt my eyes pain as I strained them downward. The Talking Stone waited for me somewhere.

And all the world seemed to wait
For some or other cause
The cause may be anything
Since when or why, who knows?

I started and woke with sleepy eyes
While I yawned and yawned
For I had to find the secret and
To wake through the day all along.

There was no shadow in the morning when the sun was in the east. For the tree stood on the path of the greater shadow of the slope, which was to its east.

The sun climbed high, burning the peeping rock on which I had taken my stand. I got up and climbed down and came near the tree. The peeping rock towered high up, throwing its own shadow on the tree. So the midday sun could not see the tree because of the peeping rock.

And the day continued with the sun riding down the west. The greater shadow of the west slope hid the tree from the softer evening light.

"Was that a secret?" I asked the sky
The sky stared back with secret eye
"Was that any secret?" I asked myself
While my foolishness I felt.

There was no need to wait there anymore. I had to tell the secret of the tree without any shadow to the Talking Stone. I had to find the Talking Stone before that. Only then could I continue my search for the big black rock from where the boat-shaped cloud would lead me to my dream, which was as impossible as glass-winged blue butterflies flying under a purple sun and orange clouds.

> So on and on I carried on
> With my loaded dream
> Till I found my way to reach
> My very impossible dream.

The dream carried me deeper into the arms of sleep where every dream was possible.

Continued Search

> I woke up to find myself
> In search of the Talking Stone
> Which somewhere lay in wait
> Hopeful and alone.

Was it morning or was it evening? I did not care anymore. For I slept and I awoke caring for time no more. Yet my heart knew one thing, better than any before: That my dream too waited, more patient than before.

Did I lose my way? I did not bother. For the entire hill looked lost and forlorn in some lost part of the world. Even birds and rock goats seemed to have been lost somewhere in some other side of anywhere. The sun must have climbed and sank. The sky too must have told yet another story, perhaps about that bush or that shallow cave. Perhaps the rolling stone rolled somewhere near or somewhere far. Nothing mattered anymore.

> All my mind thought about
> Was no fancy dream
> It thought of that blessed stone
> Knocking my thoughts within.

> Some thoughts seem to nag in mind
> With their loudest blows
> While those thoughts you wish to think
> Remain in their shadows.

So for the time being, I forgot to look for the big black rock from where the rock goat had misled me into the further misleading. I forgot about the boat-shaped cloud which would lead me to my dream, which was as impossible as glass-winged blue butterflies flying under a purple sun and orange clouds.

And then, by chance, I spotted a rock goat. The sight of it was so sudden and unexpected that I thought it to be a part of my dream. It reminded me that the big black rock was nearby. My one part of the mind argued with its another part. Should I follow the rock goat and go back to the big black rock? Or should I follow nothing and find the Talking Stone which awaited my return?

> And conflicts when turn the mind
> Into a crossroads halt,
> You wish a this, but do a that
> Then repent for the fault.

The rock goat was slowly walking across the bend. I began to follow it. With all my apologies to the Talking Stone. With all my guilt. The sky did not remind me anymore about the Talking Stone, which was waiting somewhere around. I did not look up at the sky.

Following Return

> And many a times I reasoned why
> The search for every dream
> Turns the whiles to an aimlessness
> For dreams are found within.

And dreams can scatter around also
Like those scattered stones
With each breath those dreams go out
Leaving you there alone.

On that lonely hill, I walked my way. Sometimes climbing, sometimes crawling, and all the time following the rock goat. I was careful not to lose my sight of the rock goat. Yet the thought of the Talking Stone came to me.

"Who did the Talking Stone talk to when no one around spoke?"

Again, everything in this world need not be known to you. For everything had those limitless questions following it. I was following a rock goat, for some reason which was as absurd as any impossible dream. And my dream was as impossible as glass-winged blue butterflies flying under a purple sun and orange clouds. Impossible reasons for impossible quests.

And the end question remained there with every step of mine. "What if I ever found my dream?

"And what should I follow next?"

For nothing is sure about those nexts
As sure was my step following a step
And no doubt the following of the life
With the sureness of the death.

With all those questions following me
With sure uncertainness
I knew one thing for the sure
I had to walk ahead.
No matter what or why came in
To my blessed thoughtful head
For my dream filled everything
In moments of idleness.
And whatever may be in some next
Would be my next new step
For my dream was surely hidden
In some unreachable yet.

The rock goat brought me to the foot of the hill from where I could see that road and that village. I could not see any big black rock. Everything looked possible from here.

SOME SEARCH,
SOME WAIT
AND
SOME IMPOSSIBILITY